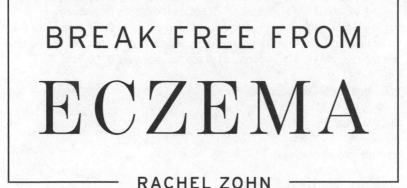

# BREAK FREE FROM
# ECZEMA

RACHEL ZOHN

*Soothe Chronic Inflammation and Itchy Skin*
*with At-Home Solutions and Proven Treatments*
*for Atopic Dermatitis*

T0022029

Published in the United States by:
Ulysses Press
P.O. Box 3440
Berkeley, CA 94703
www.ulyssespress.com

ISBN: 978-1-64604-041-4
Library of Congress Control Number: 2020931847

Printed in Canada by Marquis Book Printing
10 9 8 7 6 5 4 3 2 1

Acquisitions editor: Ashten Evans
Managing editor: Claire Chun
Editor: Anne Healey
Proofreader: Renee Rutledge
Front cover design: Hejab Malik
Cover photo: © Svetlana Lukienko/shutterstock.com

NOTE TO READERS: This book has been written and published strictly for informational and educational purposes only. It is not intended to serve as medical advice or to be any form of medical treatment. You should always consult your physician before altering or changing any aspect of your medical treatment and/or undertaking a diet regimen, including the guidelines as described in this book. Do not stop or change any prescription medications without the guidance and advice of your physician. Any use of the information in this book is made on the reader's good judgment after consulting with his or her physician and is the reader's sole responsibility. This book is not intended to diagnose or treat any medical condition and is not a substitute for a physician.

This book is independently authored and published and no sponsorship or endorsement of this book by, and no affiliation with, any trademarked brands or other products mentioned within is claimed or suggested. All trademarks that appear in ingredient lists and elsewhere in this book belong to their respective owners and are used here for informational purposes only. The author and publisher encourage readers to patronize the quality brands mentioned in this book.

# CONTENTS

# INTRODUCTION

## MY PERSONAL STORY OF ECZEMA

So what motivated me to write a book about eczema? I am a journalist and writer by trade, and in recent years I have focused on health writing. To begin with, I find that writing about health is a compelling and important topic because it's something we all care about and something we can all relate to. The well-being of our minds and bodies are deeply connected to our ability to live our best lives. Eczema is a perfect example of this, because it can have a huge impact on quality of life on many levels. I started writing about eczema several years ago, but I had no clue that I might develop the condition myself until I woke up with it one morning.

Let me just pause here to say up front that I know that my personal experience in dealing with eczema is a drop in the bucket compared with what many people have been through. This book chronicles the stories of many others who have dealt with extreme and chronic cases of eczema, and I am not one of them. But even so, eczema has left me baffled, annoyed, and frustrated. I have spent many hours combing the internet trying to figure out what the heck is wrong with my skin. And this was after I had already spent countless hours researching and writing health stories on this subject. So I can very much empathize with the plight of others who are trying to figure out this very confusing skin condition. What follows are a couple of lessons I learned the hard way.

## Eczema Can Come Back at Any Time

Like so many millions of people out there, I had eczema as a child. I'm told I had a horrible case of cradle cap as a baby. In elementary school, I had a very mild case of eczema on my hands, which basically amounted to some tiny, itchy bumps on my fingers and along my knuckles. Eventually, it went away. I honestly didn't think much about eczema for more than 35 years. Then, one morning it came roaring back with a vengeance. For unknown reasons—I hadn't used anything new on my skin or come into contact with anything irritating that I was aware of— the area around my eyelids and the area around my eyes had suddenly turned very dry and terribly itchy. The dry skin was inflamed and puffy, and over the course of a few hours, I noticed that the puffiness had created a puckered effect that created deep creases around my eyes (noticeably worse than my normal wrinkles!). The inflamed skin quickly developed into a red rash of tiny bumps.

## Eczema Is Incredibly Frustrating to Deal With

These symptoms led to my first trip to urgent care, where I received my first steroid shot. I was put on a pack of oral steroids and told to stop using any products that might have irritated my skin (I promptly threw out what I had been using). I was relieved when my symptoms quickly diminished and my face returned to normal within a day. For the next several weeks I tried to be extra careful about anything I put on my skin, but I assumed it was a one-off issue and everything would return to normal.

Except three weeks later, the same thing happened again. The same horribly itchy rash and irritated, puffy eyelids and skin returned. I ended up at a different urgent care facility and had a second steroid shot, this time coupled with a prescription for antihistamines. I was told to take the antihistamines up to three times a day for the next three weeks. I was only using a few products at this time, but I tried to cut out anything that seemed to be irritating my skin. I was even more diligent and careful about what I put on my skin.

A few weeks later when the symptoms came back yet again, I felt ready to cry. I was finally able to get an appointment to see my regular doctor, and by the time I saw him, I was feeling pretty frustrated with both my skin and the lack of information on why this was happening or what I could do to stop it. My doctor said he believed I may be experiencing a "rebound flare" from having had two steroid injections and an oral steroid prescribed within a short period of time. He prescribed tacrolimus ointment, a nonsteroidal ointment that works on the immune system, and directly on the skin cells, to suppress your skin's hyperreactive defense mechanism to irritants. It belongs to a class of drugs known as topical calcineurin inhibitors, which we'll look at more closely in subsequent chapters. I'm lucky that my insurance covered this ointment, because it's expensive.

Since then, I continue to have occasional flare-ups, and I'm usually not sure what, exactly, caused the problem. Thankfully, using a small amount of tacrolimus ointment has helped me manage these flare-ups. But to top it off, I've started to experience seborrheic dermatitis, which I have never had as an adult. And I also started to have eczema flare-ups on my hands from constant handwashing. My new beauty routine now revolves around medicated shampoos, gentle skin-care products (including some natural-base products), and thick moisturizers for my hands.

This whole experience has been eye-opening for me in terms of how difficult it is to navigate eczema treatment options to find those that will alleviate my eczema while also, hopefully, avoiding other unintended consequences. I'm still trying to figure this out for myself, just as you are, and I'm trying different things to see what works for me and what doesn't.

## We Don't Often Know Our Family History

It wasn't until after all this had happened to me that my mom told me that when she was a child, she had had a terrible case of eczema, where her hands had been so covered in a persistent, oozing eczema rash that she ended up having to halt piano lessons because she needed to keep her hands slathered in cream and wrapped tightly in gauze. She still experiences minor flare-ups when she goes through periods of stress or anxiety. I was shocked—I had never known my mom had had eczema to that extreme or that she still experiences eczema now.

It wasn't until I began to dig deeper into my research that I realized there was a hereditary link with this skin condition— if your parent had it, you have a higher chance of developing it yourself. In looking back at my own history, I realize I have several of the risk factors for developing eczema as an adult; I have a family history of it, I had eczema as a child, and I have hay fever, which I developed as a child. This certainly doesn't mean everyone with those risk factors will develop eczema. But it does offer a possible explanation as to why I was prone to developing it.

## You Aren't Alone

Here's one thing I have learned through research and my own experience: for most people, there are no easy fixes when it comes to eczema. There isn't a one-size-fits-all treatment for everyone, because what works for one person may not work for another. Finding the right treatment for you may be a matter of trial and error. Some treatments may have risks attached to them. And unfortunately, even if you have your eczema under control, and even if it's been years since you had a flare-up, it may come back at the most unexpected time. I'm sorry—that part stinks, but it's the truth. The best thing you can do is arm yourself with information, ask questions, and be willing to try different things.

You aren't alone in your frustration and anguish in coping with this condition. Maybe you've been dealing with eczema chronically since childhood. Maybe your child has eczema and you're searching for ways to help. Or maybe you're like me and this hit you out of the blue, and now you're just trying to figure out why your skin suddenly got angry and how to calm it down. Whatever the reason, you're in the right place to start your journey toward healing your skin and breaking free of eczema.

## WHY YOU NEED TO READ THIS BOOK

This book aims to empower anyone who is living with eczema or helping to care for someone with eczema to make the best choices possible for their individual skin concerns. It is not about promoting one specific treatment or perspective over another. If you are hoping for a magic cure, this isn't it because a magic cure doesn't exist, as numerous experts interviewed for this book all agree. But if you are trying to understand eczema and how you can best tackle this life-altering skin condition, this book is packed with information backed by research and expert advice.

There is a great deal of conflicting and confusing information out there on this common skin condition. This book seeks to cut through misinformation to clearly explain some of the best strategies for treating eczema, including what you can do from home and what you need to know before you see your practitioner. The overall goal of this book is to bring together a wealth of clear and accurate information so you understand your options and can make the best decisions in the care and management of your skin.

The following chapters will walk you through the ins and outs of your daily skin care regimen, including the different approaches of alternative and holistic treatments and what natural products you may want to consider trying. It also explores the link between allergies and eczema and gets you up to speed on the wave of new therapies that are on the horizon. In addition, it examines the impact that eczema has on mental, emotional, and overall health and wellness and particular concerns for patients of different ethnicities in treating eczema.

## THE EXPERT SOURCES BEHIND THIS BOOK

In researching this book, it became clear that few health books on eczema for the general public offer a cross-section of views on eczema from esteemed experts who represent contemporary medicine, cutting-edge research, holistic or alternative practices, as well as those dealing with this disease on a personal level. Aside from medical journals or medical text books, most books on this topic are primarily written from a specific viewpoint on how eczema should be treated.

A plethora of research on all aspects of eczema went into this book and serves as the foundation for the narrative, with the aim of giving readers a comprehensive understanding of eczema and making this information more accessible. This book is also the culmination of multiple interviews with 14 different experts and patient advocates who understand and live with eczema, either on a personal or professional level, or as part of their daily lives. I interviewed physicians and medical researchers, alternative and holistic practitioners, and eczema patients and parents who are dedicated to increasing awareness and furthering research on this skin condition.

Many of those I interviewed have well-developed and strong opinions about how eczema should be treated and managed. This book offers a variety of these opinions and viewpoints, along with a thorough review of what contemporary medical literature has to offer on the subject of eczema.

Lastly, please note that in an effort to keep the tone of this book more conversational and engaging, I avoided excessively referencing source material within the body of the book. I tried to judiciously include attributions to key studies, journal articles, and reports that are referenced, but please know that every part of this book is based on a combination of research and the expert opinion of those interviewed. You'll find a thorough bibliography at the back of this book.

# CHAPTER 1

# WHAT'S BEHIND YOUR ITCHY, ANGRY SKIN?

Your skin is your body's largest and heaviest organ; on average it covers 20 square feet and accounts for about 20 pounds of weight. It's an effective, waterproof covering to protect everything on the inside, including your bodily systems and internal organs, by keeping out all the things that would otherwise harm you. It plays a vital role in maintaining your immune system, regulating body temperature, and keeping water and moisture in. But your skin isn't just a fleshy barrier between your insides and the elements; it's also one of your defining and most visible features. Your skin is your exterior to the world, so when something goes wrong with it, it's sure to impact you on a number of levels. Your skin also functions as an enormous sensor that allows you to interact with the world around you. Through your skin, you feel sensations such as hot, cold, smooth, rough, pain, and that prickly, crawly, irritating sensation called itchiness.

If you have eczema, you know itchiness all too well. An eczema itch isn't a fleeting tingly or ticklish sensation. Eczema often causes a deep, agonizing, unrelenting, overwhelming irritation of the skin, and no amount of scratching, rubbing, or clawing will satisfy it. As if that's not awful enough, eczema comes with a host of other issues, causing your skin to become dry, red, cracked, bumpy, and scaly. It can leave your skin as rough as sandpaper and covered in a crust of flakes, or blotchy with weeping sores. In fact, the word eczema comes from a Greek word meaning "to boil over," which is a good way to describe the red, inflamed, and painful skin caused by this condition.

Eczema affects over 31 million people in the US—or roughly 10 percent of the population—with symptoms ranging from mild to moderate to severe, according to the National Eczema Association (NEA), a nonprofit organization dedicated to informing and educating people on this skin disease. Eczema isn't contagious, so you can't catch it by coming into contact with someone who has it, but the broken skin or deep cracks that can form with eczema can leave you vulnerable to other infections. There is no cure for eczema, so treatment focuses on managing the symptoms, helping the affected skin heal, and preventing flare-ups.

Doctors aren't sure exactly what causes eczema, but they believe that a number of factors come into play. Researchers believe that people with eczema may have abnormalities in their skin barrier, where their skin becomes "leaky" and lets in more environmental substances, such as bacteria, pollens, molds, chemicals, and other potential allergens or irritants. Research has also shown that a gene variation may affect your skin's ability to provide protection against those environmental factors, and this may trigger a reaction. People with eczema tend to have a hyperreactive immune system, so that when their skin senses a foreign substance outside or inside the body, it responds by producing inflammation.

Some people find their eczema goes away over time, but for others, it's a lifelong battle. For those people, eczema is a chronic condition that can come and go in what are known as "flare-ups" or simply "flares," where eczema symptoms are made worse by something internal, inside your body, or external, in your environment. An eczema rash can erupt on a small patch of skin, or it can sweep across large areas of your body.

If you have dealt with eczema, you probably know all too well how difficult it can be to sleep or focus on a task during a flare and how upsetting and embarrassing it can be when you see your red, inflamed skin in the mirror or on your body. Eczema can have a huge impact on your everyday life, and it's also linked to an increase in anxiety and depression. More than a third of people with eczema have reported that they "often" or "always" feel angry or embarrassed by their appearance, according to NEA.

## WHO IS AT RISK FOR GETTING ECZEMA?

A number of studies have shown that eczema is more common in people who have a family history of it, so if other relatives have eczema, you or your children may have a greater chance of developing it. People with allergies, such as hay fever, asthma, or food allergies, also have an increased risk for developing it. Up to 60 percent of people with eczema will develop asthma or hay fever later in life, and up to 30 percent have food allergies, according to the National Institutes of Health, which is part of the US Department of Health and Human Services and the nation's medical research agency.

Some people think of eczema as a childhood affliction as it's more common in children than adults, but eczema can occur at any age. According to the American College of Allergy, Asthma & Immunology, 60 percent of patients begin experiencing eczema symptoms by age one, and another 30 percent begin experiencing symptoms by age five. It's been estimated that most people will outgrow eczema before adulthood, but some studies have found that up to 80 percent may continue to have eczema symptoms into their twenties.

Cases of eczema also appear to be increasing in the population as a whole. Some studies have found that the prevalence of eczema has been increasing in the last several decades. Although it's not clear why, the American Academy of Pediatrics has found that more children are visiting their doctors for eczema, and the American Academy of Dermatology reports that more children and adults are developing eczema than ever before.

For many children, eczema takes the form of an itchy red rash of tiny bumps on their cheeks, forehead, or scalp. The rash may spread to their arms or legs or across their chest. In adults, eczema typically takes on a slightly different appearance, with the skin tending to be extremely dry and scaly. With chronic eczema, years of scratching can cause the skin to be thick and leathery, and it may have a darker or lighter appearance than the surrounding skin.

# TYPES OF ECZEMA

Eczema is a general term used to describe a group of conditions known as dermatitis, which means inflammation of the skin. There are a number of different types of eczema, and it's even possible to have more than one type on different areas of your body. It can be difficult to distinguish between various types of eczema, and each person may experience eczema a little differently. For the most part in this book, "eczema" will be used as a general term. However, it's important to get a feel for the different types of eczema, because each can have slightly unique symptoms and triggers and some types may have specific treatments.

## Atopic Dermatitis

Atopic dermatitis (also known as AD) is the most common type of eczema. According to NEA, an estimated 10 percent of all people worldwide are affected by this condition at some point in their life and more than 18 million American adults are impacted. AD often appears as a red, itchy rash that is chronic and inflammatory and often begins in childhood. Though the exact cause of AD is unknown, researchers believe that a combination of genetics and other factors are involved. AD is often triggered when the immune system goes into overdrive in response to an allergen or irritant inside or outside the body.

Atopic dermatitis tends to run in families. If one parent has AD, asthma, or hay fever, there's about a 50 percent chance that their child will have at least one of these conditions, according to NEA. If both parents have one or more of these conditions, the chances are even greater that their child will also have it. AD in adults is often a chronic condition, affecting nearly any area of the body, and for many the itching is unbearable.

Common symptoms of atopic dermatitis include the following:

• Itching
• Dry, scaly skin
• Redness
• Open, crusted, or weepy sores, especially during a flare-up

# Contact Dermatitis

Contact dermatitis happens when the skin touches irritating substances or allergens, causing it to become inflamed and turn red; it may also burn and itch. Contact dermatitis usually appears on the hands or on other parts of the body that touched the irritant/allergen, but it can be hard to distinguish from other rashes or forms of eczema. There are several kinds of contact dermatitis, the most common being irritant contact dermatitis and allergic contact dermatitis.

**Irritant contact dermatitis** occurs when the skin is repeatedly exposed to a mild irritant over a period of time. With irritant contact dermatitis, the skin can blister, crack, swell, or form open sores or ulcerations. If the skin has a wound on it, or if you have active atopic dermatitis, it's much easier for irritants to get through the skin barrier and cause irritant contact dermatitis. Common irritants include detergents, soaps, cleaners, waxes, and chemicals.

**Allergic contact dermatitis** occurs when your skin becomes sensitive to something it has previously been exposed to. You may become allergic to something you have been exposed to just once or for many years. This causes a delayed skin reaction that typically develops 12 to 72 hours after exposure. The reaction may be limited to the site of original contact, but often it spreads. The skin becomes red, hot, and itchy, and it may "weep."

Common sources of allergic contact dermatitis include metals (such as nickel), fragrances, cosmetics, topical medications, preservatives, sunscreens, and rubber ingredients.

Symptoms of contact dermatitis include the following:

- Redness and rash
- Burning or itching that may be intense but may not involve visible skin sores
- Swelling of the skin
- Intermittent dry, cracking, scaly patches of skin
- Blisters that may weep or crust over
- Stiff, tight-feeling skin

## Seborrheic Dermatitis

Seborrheic dermatitis (also known as cradle cap or dandruff) usually appears in areas where there are a lot of oil-producing glands. It is most common on the scalp, but it can also appear on the face (including the sides of the nose, around the eyebrows, behind the ears, and around the eyelids) as well as the upper chest and back. When babies get it, it's known as cradle cap; it causes crusty, scaly patches on the scalp, but it can also develop in the diaper area and look similar to a diaper rash. Cradle cap typically isn't itchy, and it usually disappears by the time a child turns one year old.

In adults, seborrheic dermatitis often takes the form of dandruff, but it can also appear on the face and in the folds of the skin. This condition can be itchy and recurrent throughout life. Unlike some other forms of eczema, seborrheic dermatitis isn't the result of an allergy. Doctors believe that genes and hormones play a role in how this condition develops and that microorganisms such as yeast that naturally live in your skin's oils may also contribute to it. Researchers believe that seborrheic dermatitis in babies may be triggered in part by hormones from the mother.

People with certain diseases that affect the immune system, such as HIV/AIDS, or the nervous system, such as Parkinson's disease, are believed to have an increased risk of developing seborrheic dermatitis. Flare-ups are more common when the weather turns cold and dry, and stress can also be a trigger. It is slightly more common in men than women.

Common symptoms of seborrheic dermatitis include the following:

- White or yellowish crusty flakes or scaly patches of skin that may look oily or waxy
- Red skin surrounded by pink patches, particularly in skin folds
- Greasy, swollen skin

## Nummular Eczema

Nummular eczema (also called nummular dermatitis or discoid eczema) is known for its distinct, coin-shaped sores, which may be smaller than 1 inch or larger than 4 inches. The rash often starts as tiny, reddish spots and blisters that ooze, according to the American Academy of Dermatology. The sores then enlarge to form coin-shaped patches, which can be very itchy. This type of eczema may be harder to treat than other types and is believed to be triggered by an injury to the skin, such as a burn, abrasion, insect bite, or dry skin in the winter. Men are more prone to nummular eczema than women, with most men being between 55 and 65 years old when they have their first outbreak. When women do get it, they tend to be younger, usually teenagers or young adults.

Some symptoms of nummular eczema include the following:

- Round, coin-shaped patches
- Itching
- Dry, scaly skin
- Wet, open, weeping sores

## Dyshidrotic Eczema

Dyshidrotic eczema (also called dyshidrosis or foot-and-hand eczema, among other names) produces small and intensely itchy deep-set blisters on the fingers, toes, palms, and soles of the feet.

You're at higher risk of developing dyshidrosis if you have a family history of it, if you have a history of atopic or contact dermatitis, or if you receive immunoglobulin infusion (usually for an immune deficiency). Triggers may include increased stress; allergies such as hay fever; frequently moist or sweaty hands and feet; and exposure to certain substances, such as nickel (used in metal-plated jewelry), cobalt (found in metal-plated objects and in pigments used in paints and enamels), and chromium salts (used in the manufacturing of cement, mortar, leather, paints, and anticorrosives).

Symptoms of dyshidrotic eczema include the following:

- Small, fluid-filled blisters (vesicles) on the fingers, hands, and feet
- Itching
- Redness
- Flaking
- Scaly, cracked skin
- Pain

# Stasis Dermatitis

Stasis dermatitis (also called gravitational dermatitis, venous eczema, and venous stasis dermatitis) is a condition that usually affects individuals who have poor circulation. It typically occurs in the lower legs, affecting one or both legs, according to the American Academy of Dermatology. As we age, the one-way valves in our veins that help push blood up the legs can stop working properly, which can lead to blood pooling in the lower extremities; this is called venous insufficiency.

Those over the age of 50 are most at risk of developing it. Swelling around the ankles is usually the first sign of stasis dermatitis, which may clear when you sleep, only to return the next day. Treatment and self-care can prevent this condition from becoming severe. This may include wearing a compression stocking and elevating your legs as needed.

The common symptoms of stasis dermatitis include the following:

- Swelling around the ankles
- Dry, cracked, scaly skin
- Itching
- Pain
- Red- to violet-colored open sores or ulcers on the lower legs or tops of the feet
- Shiny skin

# CHAPTER 2

# BEGINNING THE HEALING PROCESS

If there is one thing that people with atopic eczema can usually commiserate over, it's how incredibly hard it is to manage and control this condition. Eczema is frustratingly hard to treat because it's often difficult (or impossible) to determine what may be triggering it; sometimes we can't avoid a trigger even if we do know about it, and our triggers can change over time. Not only that, but the effectiveness of treatments can also vary from person to person and even wane over time, so what worked for years and years can sometimes stop working. In a nutshell, chronic eczema is a beast to conquer, but it can be done.

Chances are that by now you've turned to the internet and typed in a variation of "how to treat eczema," "how to prevent eczema," or "how to control eczema." And you have likely found numerous websites overflowing with advice and guidance on what works and what doesn't. For the most part, it all comes down to various methods for controlling itching and inflammation, maintaining skin health, and promoting healing while avoiding things that cause your eczema to flare.

If you have spent any time digging into the overwhelming mounds of information available out there, you've likely found not only an abundance of different treatments but that each treatment comes with pros and cons. For nearly every eczema treatment ever formulated or developed—whether through conventional medicine, natural therapies, or new and advanced treatments—there is often conflicting and confusing information about how well it works. Why is this? For a disease as confusing as chronic eczema, there is one simple truth: no one thing can fix this skin condition, because what works for some people won't work for others. And even if you do find something that works, there's no guarantee that it will always continue to be an effective treatment for you.

With that in mind, here's the basic breakdown for eczema treatments:

- There are conventional methods, which focus on evidence-based approaches to healing eczema.

- There are alternative or complementary treatments, which focus on using natural ingredients.

- There are mind-body practices, which focus on the interactions between the brain, the body, and behavior and how all three affect the body's ability to function and maintain health and well-being.

- There are integrative approaches, which seek to marry conventional and complementary treatments.

Much of this book will focus on deepening your understanding of eczema and learning about things you can do at home to better manage and treat it. But first, let's cover the basics of all of these different treatment options, so you can make well-informed decisions about what is right for you.

# GETTING THE RIGHT DIAGNOSIS: BEING SEEN AND HEARD BY YOUR DOCTOR

The first step in finding the right treatment for eczema is to first make sure you have an accurate diagnosis, and this means seeing a doctor. Don't try to self-diagnose your own eczema. If you believe you may have chronic eczema, it's important that you get your diagnosis confirmed, and the same goes if you believe your child has eczema, says Dr. Peter Lio, who was interviewed over email for this book. Lio is a clinical assistant professor of dermatology and pediatrics at Northwestern University Feinberg School of Medicine and the founding director of the Chicago Integrative Eczema Center. Lio is also a board member and Scientific Advisory Committee member of the National Eczema Association. His clinical practice is at Medical Dermatology Associates of Chicago.

It's important to get a diagnosis because a number of other skin diseases and skin reactions can mimic eczema, and there are many different types of eczema (as we saw in the previous chapter). Without an accurate diagnosis, it's much harder to treat your skin condition, explains Lio. Your primary care provider is a good place to start. Because eczema affects so many children, pediatricians see many of these cases, and most are astute in being able to diagnose and treat it, Lio says.

Your doctor will look at your symptoms, your medical and family history, and what seems to trigger outbreaks. There is an overwhelming amount of information out there about eczema, and your doctor can help you sort through what applies to you or your child and what doesn't. Before your appointment, take a moment to write down issues or concerns. This can help you make the most of your time with the doctor and ensure you have a productive discussion in which you have a chance to ask all of your questions.

# TREATMENTS TO MEND HARD-TO-HEAL SKIN

The goal with any eczema treatment is to control the itch, calm the skin from irritation and inflammation, and help the skin heal. Accomplishing this is a matter of dealing with three major hurdles, says Lio:

- Getting your skin clear
- Keeping it clear (while avoiding overuse of medication)
- Finding ways to keep that up over time

The last two can be especially challenging. This is because, while you may go through brief periods where your skin seems to calm down, before long it seems like it's flaring again, and often you have no idea why. So the next step is to know all of your treatment options and what tools are available to consistently keep it clear. For most people, it will take a combination of treatments to manage their symptoms. The question is, what will work best for you?

The first step in any eczema treatment is regular use of a good moisturizer. This is considered an essential part of treating eczema because it helps strengthen the skin barrier, Lio says. For the mildest cases, simply using a good moisturizer on a regular basis can help strengthen the skin barrier, and for a lucky few, this alone may be enough to break the itch-scratch cycle, explains Lio. This cycle is when an itch evokes the behavior of scratching, which then increases inflammation of the skin and leads to more itching, which leads to more scratching. We'll look more at how to pick moisturizers and other products that won't irritate your skin in the next chapter. However, most people with chronic eczema will need more than a good daily moisturizer, especially during flare-ups.

## Topical Steroids: A Mainstay in Treatment

Traditionally, most doctors begin treating eczema with corticosteroid creams or ointments; these are also called topical corticosteroids or topical steroids. Topical corticosteroids are applied directly to the area that is flaring to relieve inflammation and calm itching. Lio describes topical corticosteroids as the mainstay of eczema treatment: "They are inexpensive, work reliably and very quickly, and when used appropriately are very safe," Lio explains.

Hydrocortisone is a type of corticosteroid that is commonly used to treat a number of skin ailments and can be purchased over the counter in a 1 percent concentration. There are also a number of prescription topical steroids that come in varying strengths. However, topical steroids should generally be avoided in certain situations, such as eczema flares on the face. And topical steroids shouldn't be used continuously, because doing so can lead to potentially severe side effects. Lio's rule of thumb is that topical steroids shouldn't be applied to any given area for longer than two weeks per month. Keep in mind, this goes for all steroids. Even a 1 percent hydrocortisone cream isn't meant to be used on a continuous basis.

In recent years, the issue of topical steroid overuse has been gaining more recognition, with some patients rallying to raise awareness about a condition called topical steroid withdrawal or red skin syndrome. This condition has been reported in those who have used topical steroids on a long-term basis. Symptoms include extremely red, irritated skin that itches and feels like it's burning. This is a controversial and hotly debated topic within the eczema community (we'll look at it more closely in later chapters). But it's important to understand that if topical steroids aren't controlling your eczema when used in a proper manner, it may be time to think outside the box and try different treatments, Lio says.

Oral steroids, such as prednisone, are sometimes used to get a severe case under control, but many doctors believe that it is best to avoid these types of drugs if possible. This is because oral prednisone has many side effects and can even cause a rebound flare-up that is sometimes worse than where the patient began, Lio explains.

Other options that have long been used to treat very acute flares include wet-wrap therapy, which can be done with or without topical steroids. This can be done at home, often at night before bed. Wet wraps can be applied after bathing and moisturizing. With this method, you use a clean cotton cloth or gauze, which is moistened until slightly damp and wrapped around the affected area, followed by a dry dressing. Wearing this overnight or for several hours can help rehydrate and calm the skin. Lio says that some people find this therapy to be amazingly helpful.

## Nonsteroidal Medicines and New Treatment Options

An alternative to topical steroids is nonsteroidal prescription medications, such as calcineurin inhibitors and crisaborole. These can give you longer periods of anti-inflammatory treatment without using topical steroids, Lio explains. Neither of these drugs should be used on children younger than two years old.

Crisaborole is in a class of medications called phosphodiesterase inhibitors that work by blocking the action of a certain natural substance in the body that can cause inflammation. Calcineurin inhibitors work with the immune system by blocking chemicals that can cause flares. Some patients are wary of calcineurin inhibitors because this medication comes with a "black box warning," which is a public health advisory regarding safety concerns associated with the use of a drug. With this medication, the specific warning is that there is a risk that the drug could cause cancer such as lymphoma or skin cancer. However, the American Academy of Allergy, Asthma & Immunology has concluded that the risk-to-benefit ratios of these topical drugs are similar to other conventional treatments, Lio notes.

Many new therapeutic options are now being offered to people with difficult-to-control cases of chronic eczema. New treatments include systemic immunosuppressants and biologic agents such as dupilumab, explains Lio. Eczema is often a result of the immune system overreacting to a trigger—or something in our environment that causes symptoms such as inflammation. An immunosuppressant can be used to reduce this reaction and stop the itch-scratch cycle. Dupilumab (also known by the brand name Dupixent) is a biologic that works by stopping the action of certain substances in the body that cause the symptoms of eczema. This drug is given by injection to treat adults and adolescents 12 years or older with moderate to severe eczema that hasn't been controlled through topical therapies.

Another option that may be considered as a "second-line treatment" if topical therapies don't work is phototherapy (or light therapy), which uses ultraviolet light waves (a spectrum found in sunlight and also produced artificially). Phototherapy has been around for decades, but advancements in technology have improved this therapy.

In addition to standard eczema treatments, some doctors have also begun to incorporate antibacterial therapy into patients' treatment regimens. "We now realize that Staphylococcus aureus is playing a role in many patients with eczema, and seems to be the driving factor in at least some cases," Lio says. With some of his patients, Lio has used a compound approach similar to that developed by Dr. Richard Aron, a dermatologist based in South Africa. Aron's treatment regimen uses a topical steroid, a topical antibiotic, and a moisturizer. Some people have found Aron's course of treatment to be very helpful, but as is the case with many eczema treatments, there are a number of pros and cons and varying opinions about this approach.

## FIGHTING ECZEMA NATURALLY

Many people are seeking more options for managing their health, leading to growing interest in nontraditional medicines and treatments. Some people have grown leery of using too many prescription drugs and are looking for a more natural approach to treat what ails them. In treating eczema, there is often an emphasis on using products with simple ingredients; such products are usually gentler on your skin, so they may promote healing with fewer side effects. Because we still can't explain why people get eczema and there isn't a cure for it, some people are concerned that treatments using synthetic ingredients may be counterproductive or may not be fully supporting the body's natural healing processes.

A number of alternative or complementary treatments for eczema focus on incorporating natural products with lifestyle changes to manage or prevent eczema flares. These remedies include using natural substances such as aloe vera gel or coconut oil to moisturize the skin, using honey or tea tree oil for their antibacterial and anti-inflammatory effects to help heal the skin, or using apple cider vinegar or bleach diluted in a bath to fight bacteria and help heal the skin and restore a healthy microbiome (the community of microorganisms, including "good bacteria," that live on and in the body) to the skin's surface.

Lio has long been interested in alternative medicines and natural treatments, and he began looking at ways to incorporate these into his practice as far back as his medical school days. He has seen how incorporating complementary treatments can benefit many people. In fact, this is one of his favorite topics to discuss and write about, he says. "What I find is that almost everyone can use some integrative approaches: for the milder cases, sometimes alternatives can be all they need, while in more severe cases, complementary treatments can support and augment what they are doing from a conventional perspective," Lio explains. "Some of my favorites are coconut oil, sunflower oil, vitamin B12 topically applied, oral hemp oil, and black tea compresses."

He favors using an integrative approach with his patients, which means he looks for ways to incorporate complementary treatments and natural products along with more mainstream approaches and medicines. He tries to use the best of both worlds to come up with solutions that keep chronic eczema at bay. However, there are still many unanswered questions when it comes to using natural and complementary treatments, and it's important to understand that even if something is considered an alternative treatment, it can have very real pharmacological side effects. It's important to keep your doctor informed if you are using these treatments, Lio says.

# FOCUSING ON THE MIND
# AND BODY AS A WHOLE

In addition to natural treatments, alternative therapies also include mind and body practices that focus on how the brain, body, mindset, and behaviors can greatly influence wellness. Meditation techniques, posture, breathing, and relaxation can all have huge impacts on health.

Incorporating mind-body therapies can be particularly helpful in breaking the itch-scratch cycle. A mind-body therapy can help alter persistent scratching and picking, and it can be an important part of an integrative approach to treating any condition, including eczema.

When it comes to using different treatments, it's important to understand that you may need to try a number of options, and different combinations of things, to find what really works for you, notes Lio. "I will work with acupuncturists, Traditional Chinese Medicine doctors, hypnotherapists, and nutritionists to help with complex cases or for patients who are more interested in such an approach." Lio also tries to use what he really thinks will help patients and tries to minimize approaches that are not well-substantiated.

# FINDING YOUR TRIGGERS:
# THE ECZEMA "HOLY GRAIL"

When you're living with chronic eczema, you may find yourself constantly keeping track of the things you come in contact with and taking note of chemicals or substances that you believe you may react to. Everything from what type of detergent or soap you use, to changes in weather and seasons, to the type of fabric or dyes used in your clothing can be a trigger for eczema. Trying to figure out what is setting off your skin and trying to avoid possible triggers are often the most frustrating parts of having eczema. "This is one of our toughest areas, a 'holy grail' if you will. We'd love to find those triggers and make the eczema simply vanish!" Lio explains. "However, I'd argue that if one or even a few things were really behind the whole condition, then—by definition—it wouldn't actually be atopic dermatitis!"

In fact, atopic eczema, by definition, has a multitude of triggers that can make flare-ups occur. A few common triggers that affect many patients with chronic, atopic eczema include allergens such as pollen, weeds, molds, ragweed, pet dander, pet saliva, cold and dry weather, hot and humid weather, sweating, stress, and exhaustion. But these triggers are not necessarily the underlying cause of eczema; they are simply some of the things that can set off a reaction in your skin. So even if you were somehow able to eliminate all known triggers, you might still have flare-ups, Lio explains. "Even if you were to be able to avoid all of these things (which is starting to sound pretty impossible, right?), I maintain that the eczema would still be there. These are largely just contributing factors," he says.

If you can figure out some of your biggest triggers and avoid them, it may help you keep your eczema under control. But with chronic eczema, it's almost never as simple as avoiding things in your environment that can trigger a flare-up, in part because your triggers can also play off one another, causing a vicious cycle. And not all triggers can be avoided, such as the weather or stress. Not only that, but trying to avoid every conceivable trigger may be enough to drive you crazy, says Ashley Wall, who has been the voice behind the blog Itchin since '87 (http://www .itchinsince87.com) and has been dealing with eczema since she was two years old. Wall shared her story and insight into eczema in a phone interview for the book.

Trying to identify triggers is a never-ending source of conversation and debate within the eczema community, says Wall, who also regularly attends conferences on the topic. She keeps an ongoing list in her mind of things that she knows will cause her skin to react, but even so, she says it's nearly impossible to know everything that will trigger her eczema. "I don't necessarily know what all my triggers are, but I do have an idea of things in my environment that can trigger it," she says.

Extreme hot or cold weather will set her skin off. If she is staying in a hotel, the type of detergent used to launder sheets and towels can cause her skin to flare, as will most fragrances. If there's a cut on her hand and she squeezes a lemon or touches something acidic, her hand will quickly break out with eczema— same thing if she touches wool. And don't get her started about what happens if she comes into contact with latex.

"I don't necessarily know what ingredients in particular will cause a flare-up, but anything fragrant will break me out," says Wall. "But I don't know how helpful it would be to know every ingredient I'm sensitive to. I can use the most basic product with three ingredients, but if it's a hot and humid day or it's cold and brutal weather, my skin will start itching no matter what. So, it won't even necessarily be the ingredients in the products."

She does keep tabs on her environment and how she is feeling overall. If she has a flare, she'll think back to what things she has come into contact with, to see if she can identify the trigger. If she believes it's something from her environment, she'll try to take a bath or shower as soon as possible.

"Overall, I try to go with the flow," Wall explains. "I'll try and control one thing and it'll be something else. So, I try not to worry about it so much. Stress can also be a trigger."

## HAVING ANOTHER CONDITION ON TOP OF CHRONIC ECZEMA

Like Wall, many people with chronic eczema also have reactions to certain chemicals or environmental substances. Some of these people might have contact dermatitis in addition to atopic eczema, says Lio. Contact dermatitis is caused when you come into contact with a substance you are hypersensitive to and it causes you to break out in a red, itchy rash. "So, a patient might get better by avoiding exposure to a chemical or substance in the environment and they will have fewer flare-ups, but they still may have atopic dermatitis," Lio explains.

If there is a concern that you may have a contact allergy to something, you can have patch testing done by an allergist. This is where a series of patches filled with potential allergens are taped to your back for two days. There is no needle-pricking involved, such as you would have with a skin prick test for hives, which is a different allergic response from eczema. A patch test cannot show what foods you could be allergic to, Lio notes. It can show whether you have a hypersensitivity reaction to certain substances, active ingredients, preservatives, or fragrances. When the patches are removed, your doctor can see what specific substances your skin is reacting to, Lio says.

He explains that one common ingredient that more people—both children and adults—have been testing positive to is an allergen called methylchloroisothiazolinone, or its close cousin methylisothiazolinone. These substances may be abbreviated as

MCI and MI in a list of ingredients. "They are both preservatives found in lots of products, including 'wet wipes' and 'baby wipes' and can cause all sorts of trouble by driving an eczema reaction," says Lio. "This does not mean that these chemicals are 'bad' per se, it just means that for some people an allergy can develop, which can then make them break out in eczema."

## CAN FOOD BE A TRIGGER?

Food is another common factor that people believe may cause eczema. In fact, Lio has seen many families who are convinced that food is the root cause of their or their child's eczema, and this is made even more complex because food allergies are definitely associated with atopic dermatitis, with up to one-third of moderate to severe patients having food allergies, Lio says. Food allergies can be potentially dangerous or life threatening for some people and are known to cause hives, angioedema, and anaphylaxis. For the majority of people with both eczema and food allergies, eating a food you are allergic to may be more apt to cause hives, Lio explains. However, according to the American Academy of Dermatology, food allergies and a flare-up of eczema don't always go hand in hand. Even with specific testing for food allergies, researchers have found that food allergies don't usually provoke immediate eczema symptoms.

In fact, new research is changing our understanding about the connection between food allergies and eczema flares, Lio says. Instead of food potentially causing eczema, it seems that eczema may actually be the cause of food allergies in some cases involving babies and young children, he explains. Researchers now believe that for some babies, a damaged skin barrier allows food proteins to abnormally enter the body, and this stimulates allergy. "This may be the most exciting development of the past few years and may give us a new understanding into what amounts to a reversal in thinking about food allergies: It is now thought that at least some food allergies (such as peanut) actually may be caused by eczema!" says Lio. "This is exciting to me because it truly takes this story of foods triggering eczema and turns it on its head."

However, this doesn't mean that food doesn't play some role in triggering eczema. Some people may have a reaction to eating certain foods. For example, for some people, eating things such as sugar, eggs, or dairy may prompt an "eczematous food reaction," which will develop sometime after eating the food, Lio says. This reaction has more to do with having a food sensitivity or intolerance to certain foods, and it can take days to manifest and is different from the immediate reaction produced by a food allergy. Also, some people find that their skin does better overall, and they have fewer eczema flare-ups, when they're off of certain foods. This may be because some foods cause an inflammatory response, Lio explains.

Another issue when it comes to food and eczema is that it's often hard to tell what symptoms are being caused by what issue. If it seems like every time you eat certain foods, your skin seems to break out with eczema, it's natural to link your eczema to eating those foods, says Zainab Danjuma, a London resident and YouTube vlogger who has had eczema since she was a baby. Danjuma, who was interviewed via video chat for this book, also has hay fever and a type of food allergy known as oral allergy syndrome.

For Danjuma, eating certain foods—such as carrots, cherries, bananas, apples, and strawberries—will cause an immediate reaction in which the inside of her mouth will start to tingle and itch and her throat will become scratchy. However, if the foods are cooked, she doesn't have this reaction. Danjuma has a stronger (although not life-threatening) reaction to peanuts: a mouthful of a peanut-based sauce will set off a full-body rash that can leave her skin irritated for days. This type of food allergy can happen to those who are allergic to pollens, because the proteins of certain raw fruits, vegetables, seeds, or nuts are similar in structure to the pollen of some trees and grasses, leading the immune system to react to these foods the same way it reacts to pollen.

Sometimes her food allergy reaction gives her hives, which may also contribute to a rashy, eczematous reaction on her skin, says Danjuma, who has opened up about her lifelong eczema affliction on her YouTube channel, IAmBeeZee. "It seems like I have a baseline of eczema, even on a good day," Danjuma says. "So, if I have hives, and it goes away, I will also have eczema, and that rash lingers much longer."

## THE ULTIMATE GOAL: BREAKING THE "VICIOUS CYCLE"

It's not uncommon for people to want to launch into potentially costly and time-consuming testing in the hopes of finding answers. Lio has seen many patients do this, but unfortunately, it rarely gives them helpful information, he says. "This includes people who have moved houses or even out of a city, state, or country, and have gotten rid of pets only to find that things seem to get right back to where they were," says Lio.

So instead of taking such drastic measures, Lio tries to focus on ways to break the vicious "itch-scratch-itch" cycle caused by eczema. He has found that the best success in managing chronic eczema comes when you can control the inflammation and itch, treat the abnormal microbiome that accompanies eczema, repair the skin-barrier damage, and manage how eczema affects the mind-body relationship. In doing this, "we find that for most of our patients, we can get the eczema under great control and give them their lives back," says Lio. "Moreover, we find that if we do this for a few months, many patients can enter a sort of remission from the eczema: a period where they find things are nice and calm, they need little or no treatment for their skin."

When you're able to put your skin into a quiet phase, where it's calmed down for an extended period of time, you've truly broken the vicious cycle. This is what Lio calls a "virtuous cycle," meaning you have a healed skin barrier, decreased inflammation, and a normalized microbiome. When you do this, you're able to get good, quality sleep and have a feeling of well-being and wholeness again.

## WHEN IT SEEMS LIKE NOTHING IS WORKING AND NO ONE IS LISTENING

But getting to that quiet phase sometimes seems unattainable. For many people, dealing with eczema is a lonely and frustrating experience that is heightened if they don't feel like they have anyone to turn to, or if they feel like no one really hears or can help them. For some, this feeling of isolation is compounded when it seems like even their doctors don't understand what's going on with their skin.

This has been the situation for Danjuma for much of her life, and she has vented about the topic in several of her YouTube videos. Like many people who struggle with eczema, Danjuma simply lost faith that her doctors really understood what she was going through. Instead, she felt like they pushed medicines on her that weren't working and that she feared might actually be making her skin worse. "Every time I applied some of these creams, my skin hurt worse. It would make me itchier and more rashy," she says. "I decided to do this by myself. I'm just too wary of going out to find someone who will listen to me."

It's been nearly a decade since she gave up on trying to get doctors to listen to her. The final straw came when, as a university student, her eczema began to flare uncontrollably, covering nearly her whole body. She wanted her doctor to see what she was going through and give her options, but that didn't happen. "I remember walking out of the room crying, and the doctor came after me and said, 'Ok, ok, we'll send you for more tests.' But all I could think was, I shouldn't have to be crying before you'll listen to me," Danjuma says.

Her doctor put in a referral for her to see a specialist, and Danjuma waited six months to be seen again. When the day of her appointment finally arrived, Danjuma felt excited that maybe this doctor would be able to give her answers or give her different treatment options. But once again, she felt hustled through the appointment, and she left feeling deflated and frustrated. "That doctor just said, 'Let me see your ankle,' and I just pulled down one edge of my sock," she says. "That was it. I had waited six months for that. He didn't even look at my back, which was very wet and oozy and the worst at that time. I was ready to strip down naked, to have swabs and blood tests; something. But he just started typing out a prescription for all the same general medicines I had tried before."

Since discussing her experiences on YouTube, Danjuma has heard from others who have had similar experiences. "I've heard people say that if they bring up their concerns, the doctor thinks you're overexaggerating or you're being a hypochondriac,"

Danjuma says. "So you end up skirting around the issue of the skin when you talk to your doctor. So, instead you'll ask them, 'What can you give me to help me sleep better at night?' because if you can get a good night's sleep, you'll feel in a better mood."

Part of the problem is that it seems like few doctors have lived with eczema themselves or have a deeper understanding of how frustrating it is to deal with chronic eczema on a daily basis, Danjuma notes. Instead, it can feel like some doctors approach their patients from a strictly clinical perspective, without seeing the patient's side.

"It's like they look at it as a simple diagnosis; if it's dry skin and it's red and itchy, it's eczema," Danjuma says. "But they don't understand the ins and outs of it. Sometimes you'll get a rash for no reason at all. You haven't done anything and it's completely random. And you tell them the cream doesn't work. But it seems like they're just looking at the textbook and saying, 'No, this is what it says to do. You just need to use more cream.'"

There are doctors out there who are willing to listen and can help, Lio says. Finding the right patient/doctor fit isn't always easy, but the first step to making sure you're being heard is to practice good communication and state as clearly as you can what your concerns are and what you want, says Lio. His advice: if you and your doctor don't click, try seeking other opinions until you find someone you feel you click with.

Press to see a specialist, such as a dermatologist or an allergist, or seek out another doctor's recommendation for treatment. "While I'd like to say that all dermatologists understand the burden of skin disease and are therefore kind and caring, well, we know that everyone is different. Sometimes, it's really a matter of fit," explains Lio.

If your case is severe and seems to be getting significantly worse over time, or your skin doesn't seem to be responding to treatment the way it should, it may be time to seek a second opinion, says Lio. "There are certainly cases I have seen that have been incorrectly diagnosed and many, many more that have been poorly managed," he says. "So, if things aren't going the way they should, it's really important to get other opinions."

# CHAPTER 3

# THE BASICS OF SKIN CARE AND UNDERSTANDING YOUR SKIN

Proper skin care is essential for skin health, whether or not you have eczema. But if you struggle with eczema, then you know how tricky skin care can be. A trip to the store to buy products may be an exercise in frustration that leaves you feeling broke and annoyed at spending money on products that don't seem to help. Faced with a sea of products that all claim to be beneficial, how do you choose the right ones? Trying to determine the best skin-care products to use can be like trying to fill in multiple-choice answers without knowing the question—you're picking something without really knowing if it's a valid solution.

When it comes to eczema, the right skin care depends on your unique skin issues and what's going on with your skin at that moment. How you treat your skin during an active flare is very different from how you treat your skin when it's stable and relatively eczema-free. When your skin is doing well, it's important that you set up a good skin-care routine that will help it stay healthy. Ultimately, this should help reduce flares and help your skin recover faster.

It may be tempting to put skin care on the back burner when your eczema has simmered down, but that's the time to implement strategies to further strengthen and bolster your skin, so you can ultimately avoid more flare-ups down the road. Think of these strategies as working to prevent the fire from erupting from within.

The first step in setting up your skin-care regimen is to make sure you're doing everything you can to maintain your skin, protect it, and avoid flare-ups, says Dr. Adam Friedman, professor and interim chair of Dermatology, Residency Program director, director of Translational Research, and director of Supportive Oncodermatology at the George Washington University School of Medicine and Health Sciences. Friedman was interviewed for this book by phone. He shared daily tips to help keep eczema skin under control.

Happy skin starts with managing your eczema through your daily skin-care regimen, so let's start with the basics.

## BUT FIRST, A QUICK SCIENCE TUTORIAL

Good skin care begins with using the right cleansers. You probably already guessed that gentle soaps and cleansers are best, but to understand why, let's take a little science refresher on pH levels. Measured on a scale of 0 to 14, pH indicates how acidic or basic (alkaline) a substance is. The measurement of pH is based on the concentration of hydrogen ions in a solution; the higher the concentration, the more acidic the solution and the lower the pH. For instance, lemon juice, which is very acidic, has a pH of about 2.

Toward the opposite end of the scale, soap, which is very alkaline, has a pH of about 12. Pure water is neutral, with a pH of 0.

The surface of the skin is known as the acid mantle, which is a very fine, slightly acidic film that acts as a barrier. For most people, this layer has a pH level of around 5. However, people with chronic eczema often have a higher-than-normal skin pH level, perhaps closer to 10. This results in your skin becoming dry and sensitive, which can exacerbate eczema and trigger inflammation and flare-ups. A higher-than-normal pH level is just one of many reasons why people with eczema have skin-barrier problems, and it basically means that your skin isn't functioning properly.

So when shopping for soaps, it's helpful to look for brands that are pH balanced. You want to avoid soaps that are too alkaline, as this can increase the skin's pH to a level that could impair the skin barrier function, Friedman says.

## THE BASICS OF BATHING: BE GENTLE

Another reason you should ditch harsher soaps is that they use surfactants, or "surface active agents," which is the key cleaning ingredient that breaks down oil and dirt on the skin, explains Friedman. "Surfactants pull dirt from the skin, but in essence they also pull some of the skin off with it," he says.

The outermost layer of the skin is designed to keep harmful stuff out, but surfactants can cause problems in skin where the outermost layer doesn't function properly. Surfactants can further weaken this defense mechanism. Some examples of common surfactants that people with eczema may find irritating are sodium lauryl sulfate (SLS), also known as sodium dodecyl sulfate (SDS), and sodium laureth sulfate (SLES), which has a similar chemical formula to SLS/SDS. These ingredients all contribute to the foaming and lathering properties of soap and cleansing products. And while they have been deemed to be safe, they are known to cause irritation in some people.

Friedman advises patients shopping for skin-care products to carefully read labels and to check out the website of the National Eczema Association. NEA recognizes products that are suitable for people with eczema and sensitive skin through its Seal of Acceptance program. The NEA Seal of Acceptance review panel examines these products, looking at the testing data on skin sensitivity as well as product ingredients and formulations. Some examples of brands that NEA includes on its list of cleansers or body washes are CeraVe, Triple Soap, CLn, Cetaphil, Honest, and Aveeno, but there are a number of other brands available.

"The unifying feature of mild soaps is that they have minimal or no surfactants in them," Friedman explains. Some products also use newer technology that prevents surfactants from penetrating into the skin, so they are less irritating and are also safe for people with eczema to use, Friedman notes.

However, even the mildest and gentlest soaps will remove some of the skin's lipids, or oily sebum and natural fats, and natural moisturizing factors. So regardless of whatever mild soap you're using, if your skin is actively flaring, "you should use zero soap, none whatsoever," says Friedman. During a flare, try showering or bathing in plain water, because it's by far the gentlest option.

## SOAK UP! THEN MOISTURIZE, MOISTURIZE, MOISTURIZE

In an ideal world, eczema patients would spend time soaking in a tub every day, long enough to get their fingers and toes wrinkly, Friedman says. This isn't always feasible, so showering is fine, but feel free to let the water run on you a little while so your skin can soak up that moisture. And when possible, a good soak in the tub will help water really seep into the top layer of skin, Friedman explains. "You really want the skin to be saturated. When the skin becomes pruney, that's how you know that water has gotten into the top layer."

However, it's best to stick to a once-a-day bath or shower and avoid steaming-hot water when bathing. That doesn't mean you have to use cool water, but a comfortable lukewarm temperature is fine and won't strip your skin of its natural oils like hot water can, Friedman explains. But the real key to bathing properly is what you do immediately after getting out of the bath or shower: slather on the moisturizer.

"You want to pat dry just a little bit and you want to put your moisturizer on damp skin," Friedman says. He recommends applying moisturizer within 30 seconds to 1 minute after getting out of the bath or shower. Doing this will help lock that moisture into your skin and help it function properly. The key is to allow just a little bit of water to evaporate off the skin, but not too much, because evaporation will quickly begin pulling water out of the skin, which will dry it out, he explains.

## UNDERSTANDING OUR SKIN'S MACHINERY

If you have chronic eczema, your skin's machinery doesn't function properly. Some people with eczema may balk at constantly using a moisturizer, in part because it may sting or hurt when it's applied to broken skin. But it's important to understand the larger role our moisturizers play in maintaining a healthy skin microbiome and helping it do its job, Friedman explains. To understand why, we have to understand how our skin works.

Our skin is divided into different layers: the first (or top) layer is the epidermis, the second layer is the dermis, and the bottom layer is made up of subcutaneous fat. New skin is made at the bottom of the epidermis, and then these skin cells travel up to the top layer and eventually flake off. The outermost layer of the epidermis is called the stratum corneum, which is made up of dead cells. People once thought that this layer was devoid of any function or biological activity, but that's not true, Friedman explains. "Even though that skin is dead, there's a lot going on there," he says.

The stratum corneum serves as the major barrier between our bodies and the surrounding environment. It protects our underlying tissues and organs from infection, dehydration, outside chemicals, and injury. This tough outer layer has been described as being like a brick wall, with cells layered together like bricks and mortared together by lipids. "There's a lot going on in this layer. There are proteins that are making the fats, which cement and keep that top layer together," Friedman explains. "There are proteins working to break apart the connection between the dead cells. And all those proteins need water to function."

So if your top layer of skin gets too dried out, it stops working correctly, Friedman says. "What you see as dry skin is actually retained dead skin that isn't being shed as it should be because your skin's machinery isn't working correctly," he explains. For people with chronic eczema, this creates skin-barrier dysfunction that leaves the skin more susceptible to environmental damage and allows allergens to penetrate through its layers. This makes the skin more vulnerable to secondary infections from bacteria, viruses, and fungi.

# THE ROLE OF NATURAL MOISTURIZING FACTORS

A key component to maintaining proper skin hydration is the natural moisturizing factors (NMF) found in the top layer of skin. These are naturally occurring humectants, which include chemicals produced by the body, such as hyaluronic acid, which work to pull water and moisture from the deeper skin layers to moisturize and protect the top layer of skin. Humectants help it maintain adequate hydration, and keep it healthy. NMF is a mix of substances that draw in atmospheric water. This is why your skin seems drier when there isn't enough humidity in the air—your skin isn't able to draw in enough moisture from the surrounding air. NMF is also an important part of keeping harmful microorganisms from invading the skin. Having low NMF in your skin is associated with more severe cases of eczema.

When you wash or rinse your face, even with just water, you lose some of these factors, Friedman says. Because people with chronic eczema already don't make enough NMF, it's crucial that they replenish these natural humectants with a good moisturizer, as this will help keep the skin healthy and the skin barrier functioning correctly, he notes.

Friedman recommends using a moisturizer that contains humectants, which work by attracting water molecules to them like a magnet—much as your natural moisturizing factors would do. A moisturizer with humectants will pull water from the deeper layer of the dermis, increasing the level of moisture in the top layer of skin. Humectants include ingredients such as glycerin, sorbitol, hyaluronic acid, urea, and sodium lactate.

# MOISTURIZING BROKEN SKIN: GOOPY VS. STINGY

Friedman also recommends using products that have silicone derivatives, such as dimethicone and cyclomethicone. These are like thin versions of Vaseline; they work to lock in moisture, and if the product also has a humectant, it will bind the water and keep the moisture in your skin, he explains.

However, if your skin is very broken and irritated, you may be reluctant to use cream moisturizers because they sting and can be uncomfortable to put on an inflamed eczema flare-up. This is one of those areas where patients have to decide what they are willing to tolerate, Friedman explains. The problem is that almost anything you put on skin that is broken or cracked, or that has fissures in it, is going to burn, because you're essentially putting a cream on an open wound.

"When your skin is flared, the nerves in your skin are already 'hyped up' and your body is more prone to secreting inflammatory factors, which can cause more itchiness, discomfort, and stinging," Friedman explains. "It's a hot mess; it's our body turning against itself. It's not autoimmune, but more like your body is doing all the wrong things."

In this situation, he asks his patients: "Do you want goopy or stingy?" You can use ointments that won't sting, but they're goopy and won't work as well as creams. But creams, because of their composites, will sting a little bit more. Putting them on when your skin is still wet from a shower or bath will also help, Friedman adds.

"Certainly, slathering yourself in plain old petroleum Vaseline goopiness will lock in the water and it will have a hydrating effect," Friedman says. "But you get more bang for your buck with creams."

## THE SKIN MICROBIOME: CREATING BALANCE FOR HEALTHY SKIN

Over the last decade, researchers have been studying the importance of the human microbiome, the collection of microorganisms (including fungi, bacteria, and viruses) that live in the gut, mouth, and various other places in the body, including the skin. This has led to increasing interest in the importance of maintaining a healthy skin microbiome, Friedman explains.

It has long been known that people with chronic eczema are more prone to skin infections, including bacterial infections from Staphylococcus aureus, fungal infections such as ringworm or tinea, and viral infections such as herpes simplex. Recent studies have found that people with eczema often have an imbalance of certain bacteria in their skin microbiome. In particular, people with severe eczema tend to have higher levels of Staphylococcus aureus (Staph. aureus, often referred to simply as "staph"), which is known to cause a host of skin infections, such as impetigo, cellulitis, folliculitis, and abscesses.

Researchers in one 2017 study supported through the National Institutes of Health (NIH) found that this strain of bacteria dominated the skin microbiome of children during severe eczema flare-ups. When the children had only mild or no symptoms, the mix of bacteria on their skin was more diverse. Another NIH study found that other types of staphylococcus bacteria on the skin produced a compound that inhibits the growth of Staph. aureus and that transplanting these bacteria could have clinical benefits. As such studies indicate, in healthy skin the various microorganisms, or microbiota, work together to balance each other out. But in patients with eczema, Staph. aureus seems to have the peculiar ability to colonize the skin, and this bacterium is often found in active eczema lesions. These findings echo research on the gut microbiome that has linked a greater diversity of gastrointestinal bacteria to better digestive health.

Researchers now believe that one important element in managing eczema is finding ways to maintain the balance of microbiota, or the microorganisms living on the skin. "We know that hundreds of different species live on the skin in different amounts, all living in harmony," Friedman explains in a phone interview. "Patients with atopic dermatitis may have a low diversity of microbiota on their skin. When the diversity of organisms goes down, certain bacterium, like staph, goes up and that decrease in diversity will actually precede an active flare."

## PREBIOTICS: THE CARE AND FEEDING OF YOUR SKIN MICROBIOTA

This is where probiotics and prebiotics come into play in skin care. When you think of probiotics, you probably think of yogurt or other fermented foods or over-the-counter supplements that are chock-full of "good" bacteria such as lactobacillus and bifidobacterium. These bacteria are associated with promoting a healthy digestive tract and a healthy immune system.

But just as important are prebiotics, which act like fertilizers to stimulate the growth of the "good" bacteria living in your gut. Prebiotics for the digestive tract include plant fibers that are found in many fruits and vegetables. These fibers aren't digestible by your body, so they pass through your digestive system, where they become food for bacteria and other microbiota. Prebiotics go hand in hand with probiotics to establish and maintain a healthy gut microbiome.

Researchers believe that the same concept is true for our skin microbiome. Moisturizers serve as prebiotics for our skin microbiota, Friedman explains. "They have minerals, carbohydrates, lipids, proteins; all of this is the fodder to support well-balanced microbiota," he says. Thus, skin-care products with the right prebiotics might be able to help rebalance the skin microbiome by feeding the "good" microbiota and decreasing the "bad" microbiota.

With this in mind, companies that make skin-care products have developed a new crop of products containing prebiotics and probiotics. Two such companies—La Roche-Posay and Aveeno—have been investing in research in this area. "Some companies are trying to be more purposeful about what's in their moisturizer," notes Friedman. "There is a good amount of evidence that certain products may be able to help decrease the few microbiota that are overgrowing and rebalance things to that person's baseline, simply by using a moisturizer."

It's hard to say which skin-care lines are the best, and there is still much to learn in this area, Friedman says. We are still a ways off from understanding what it would take to provide optimum support for a healthy skin microbiome. Friedman notes that it would require a great deal of research and study to determine the perfect combination of minerals, elements, and proteins to foster a healthy microbiota.

## BLEACH BATHS

If you or your child has eczema, chances are you have heard of bleach baths. The first time you heard about it, you might have balked—just the idea of getting your inflamed skin near anything with bleach in it probably sounded like a form of torture. But many people find that bleach baths help their symptoms, and many doctors and even natural healers recommend using them. It's important to keep in mind that bleach should always be used in very low concentrations. Friedman recommends using a quarter cup of bleach in a 40-gallon bathtub.

Bleach baths have long been recommended as a treatment for eczema because of their antimicrobial and other disinfecting properties. "We thought that because of the microbiome imbalance, that this was a way of decreasing staph on the skin and giving the skin a chance to rebalance itself," Friedman explains. However, new evidence suggests that the real benefit of bleach baths is that they produce an anti-inflammatory effect on the skin, which is also key in improving eczema.

If taking a bath isn't your thing—or maybe you only have access to a shower—there are "bleach bath in a bottle" products available that may be worth trying.

## ECZEMA SKIN THROUGH THE SEASONS

The type of climate you live in has an impact on your skin. If you live in a desert, you may find that your skin dries out very easily. If you live in a tropical environment, you know that a humid summer brings a host of other issues, because sweltering temperatures and sweat can also be irritating to the skin.

But generally, weather in the winter tends to be dry, leaving your skin extra parched and vulnerable to flare-ups, Friedman explains. Also, certain fabrics, such as wool (which contains a naturally occurring wax called lanolin), can be very irritating and will easily cause your skin to feel itchy, according to Friedman.

In the winter it's important to wear protective, long-sleeved clothing made of nonirritating fabric, such as 100 percent cotton or silk. "When it's cold and windy out, try to cover up as much as possible as that will limit how much the wind dries out your skin," he explains.

Also, don't be afraid of getting some sun, especially when the weather is good. That doesn't mean you should go outside without sunscreen or allow yourself to get burned, but sunlight in moderation is known to help eczema, Friedman explains. The ultraviolet (UV) rays in sunlight can help suppress overactive immune system cells in the skin that cause inflammation. This is the basic principle behind phototherapy, or light therapy, which uses artificially produced UV light to treat eczema.

However, if you're going to be outside for more than a few minutes, don't forget the sunscreen. Friedman recommends using mineral-based sunscreens, with ingredients such as zinc oxide or titanium dioxide, because they are better tolerated and tend to be less irritating to the skin than chemical sunscreens.

## EXERCISE AND ECZEMA

If you know you're going to be doing something active, Dr. Friedman suggests wearing wicking clothes. Moisture-wicking material moves sweat to the fabric's outer surface so that it evaporates rapidly instead of saturating the fabric. This not only prevents the discomfort of having wet, sticky clothing against your skin but also helps keep you cool by allowing the sweat to evaporate from your skin. If you can, wash up as soon as you're done with the activity, even if it's just a quick rinse in plain water. If that's not an option, towel off or use a wet washcloth to remove the sweat, followed by a moisturizer. Doing this will limit sweat-associated irritation, Friedman explains.

He also recommends wearing cotton underwear and undergarments. You can also use a barrier cream like zinc oxide to protect "hot spots" on your skin or places you're more likely to experience a flare during exercise, Friedman says. A barrier cream will repel water and sweat and can be especially helpful in folds of the skin.

Peter Tapao, a fitness professional from the San Francisco Bay Area, has lived with eczema his whole life and shared his exercise tips during a phone interview for this book. (I will cover more of Tapao's personal story on page 64.) Tapao recommends keeping several spare workout shirts with you, so that you can change immediately after a workout, or even in the middle of a workout if you get too sweaty. Pat yourself down with an absorbent towel frequently during workouts. If you have hand eczema, try wearing workout gloves or yoga grip gloves that cover as much of your hands as possible.

Let yourself rest and cool down between sets or when there is a break in a class. And while you want to stay as dry as possible during exercise, avoid working out in front of a fan, which may only dry out your skin more, Tapao explains. However, if he gets itchy or feels like his skin is drying out during a workout, he'll use a spray bottle filled with spring water to spray on his face or whatever area is feeling irritated. He has found that a light spray of water keeps his skin feeling moisturized and keeps sweat from irritating his skin. He waits to apply creams or heavier ointments until after he showers, when they will absorb more easily into his skin.

Other fitness tips Tapao recommends for people with eczema:

- Don't feel like you have to work out intensely for a long period of time. Break up your exercise into increments to keep yourself from getting overly sweaty, which can cause itchiness and irritation. Start out by doing 15 minutes, but make that time count by focusing on form and building strength.

- If aerobic exercise and sweat cause your skin too many problems, try doing yoga or simply stretching. You can also do body-weight exercises, which focus on building strength and flexibility by using your body weight for resistance. These include lunges, planks, squats, leg lifts, push-ups, and more. Whenever you have to hold a pose for a period of time, you are building strength and burning calories without necessarily causing your body to overly heat up, Tapao says.

- Don't forget to drink plenty of water during your workout. This will keep you hydrated from the inside.

## TIPS AND TRICKS TO IMMEDIATELY SOOTHE THE ITCH

If you need immediate relief from an itch, there are a few things you can try doing to calm the itch down instead of raking your nails over your skin. Here are a few tips from Friedman and Rebecca Bonneteau, a naturopath who specializes in helping people with eczema (I will cover more of Bonneteau's personal story, as well as her expertise in natural and alternative treatments for patients with eczema, in Chapter 6 and Chapter 7).

- Try using cold packs or icing the area, advises Friedman. Similar nerves transmit temperature sensations and itch and pain sensations, so you can overwhelm the itch with something cold.

- Try pushing down and applying pressure to the itchy area, as this may help squelch the itch, says Bonneteau.

- Mix some peppermint essential oil with coconut oil and apply that to the skin, as this has a cooling effect on the skin that can dull the itch, says Bonneteau.

- Try crushing basil leaves in your hand and rubbing them on the area of the skin that itches, Bonneteau recommends.

- Dead Sea mud is messy but can offer relief by helping the skin cool down, Bonneteau advises. Dead Sea mud is harvested from the mineral-rich Dead Sea, a small body of water nestled in the Jordan Rift Valley between Israel to the East and Jordan. The geographical features of the Dead Sea—including the fact that the lake is at the lowest sea level of any body of water on Earth—makes the surrounding silt and mud rich with a unique combination of minerals like magnesium, sodium, and potassium. The magnesium in Dead Sea salt has also been shown to help reduce itchiness and reduce skin redness.

- If all else fails, look for distractions. Sometimes it helps to keep your hands busy or find something else to focus on. If you can take your mind off the itch, you can break the itch-scratch cycle, Bonneteau says.

# CHAPTER 4

# PERSONAL STORIES AND STRATEGIES FOR LIVING WELL WITH ECZEMA

If you have chronic eczema, chances are the state of your skin is never far from your mind. When you live with eczema, it sometimes seems like your skin condition takes precedence over everything else. It might mean that you feel like you have to think through your activities well in advance, deciding what you and your skin are up to handling that day and what might be best to avoid.

So how do you embrace life and find ways to do all the things that bring you joy while also maintaining the health of your skin? You don't want to stop doing all of your favorite activities for fear you're going to end up in an eczema flare. If you're constantly putting your life on hold, you're losing out on so many activities and interactions that can bring you fulfillment, and you're missing out on making so many memories.

Every person who deals with chronic eczema will likely face these issues again and again. Hopefully you'll come up with your own unique strategies to live your life even when your skin isn't the best. But sometimes we all need a little inspiration. Here are three stories of people who shared their strategies for living their best life and maintaining their sanity, even when their skin was driving them crazy.

## ASHLEY LORA:
## Put Yourself into a Healing Mindset

After years of dealing with eczema, Ashley Lora not only learned to reclaim her life but also found the courage to share her struggles on national television and to launch a movement to help others create their best life. Lora, who considers herself a wellness entrepreneur, is the founder of VisionHERy, a movement dedicated to empowering women. She shared her story of how her battle with eczema eventually helped her embrace her inner strength during a phone interview for this book.

Lora understands all too well the power that eczema can have over someone. She has dealt with this skin condition her whole life, often missing days of schools when her skin would flare horribly. She spent years hiding her skin, ashamed of what she looked like and also constantly worrying about everything she came into contact with and how it would affect her skin. She lived her life being cautious about what clothes she wore, because certain fabrics irritated her skin, and what foods she ate, because her food allergies seemed to trigger eczema flares.

Years later, as an adult, Lora realized that she had let her eczema take center stage in her life. "Everything I did—where I went, what I wore, who I was with—it all centered around eczema," she says. "And what a transition it was when I took eczema out of the center and put myself back in."

It's been a long road to healing, but Lora attributes much of her ability to break free from eczema to having a "healing mindset practice." For Lora, the basis of this practice is to first be well aware of her emotions and how they are influencing her. She has noticed that while things in her environment can trigger her eczema, one of the biggest triggers is her own emotions.

"Anytime I'm feeling stressed out, angry, frustrated, or if I have resentment toward another person, basically any emotion that is not good or joyful or loving, I will get a flare," Lora explains. "I realized that when I released that energy and let go of whatever was causing my emotions to not be joyful and loving, my eczema goes away. I wish I was kidding when I say right away, but it's like an immediate change."

When she realizes that there is something bothering her, she begins doing something that immediately brings her peace and calms her down. This includes practicing meditation, writing in her journal, reading the Bible, or praying. "My eczema symptoms don't exist on the conscious level when I am joyful, loving, and peaceful," Lora says.

Her journey to healing began after she graduated from college in 2014, when she experienced the most severe eczema flare of her adult life. She went back to her old standby of relying heavily on topical steroids to treat her skin, but they weren't working. Through a mound of research, she learned about topical steroid addiction and withdrawal, and suddenly things clicked. She had been using topical steroids to treat her skin for over 20 years, and, she realized, they were starting to do more harm than good. She decided it was time to discontinue her use of topical steroids.

Going through topical steroid withdrawal was a painful and exhausting process that left her looking like a snake, with peeling skin, Lora says. She kept a vacuum by her bed for the skin she was constantly shedding. She would lay in bed and visualize her life after she had healed, wearing shorts and having fun. About eight months after starting the withdrawal process, she was accepted into a clinical trial for dupilumab (now sold under the brand name Dupixent), a targeted biologic therapy administered by injection.

During that time, Lora's skin was able to heal, and she had clear skin for the first time in her life. By the summer of 2016, she was ready to celebrate by wearing shorts as often as she could—a first for her. "Even that winter, when I went home to New York to see my family, I would wear shorts to the gym, even though it was snowing outside," Lora says with a laugh. "There was no way I was hiding my legs."

She also began creating vision boards to help herself clearly visualize her goals for the coming year. One of her main goals was getting on television to share her story. In early 2018 she was a guest on the TV show *Dr. Phil*, where she laid bare her struggles with eczema and the toll it had taken on her self-esteem. She also launched VisionHERy and started holding workshops and doing speaking engagements to help others create and embrace their own goals and visions for their future.

Lora is now off of Dupixent and manages her skin condition largely with natural products. Her message to others is to visualize your future and then move toward your goals.

"Many people with eczema hesitate or stop doing what they want to do, simply because they're too afraid their eczema may flare," Lora says. "My advice: Do it anyways and handle the consequences later, if it even shows up. Make your eczema your best friend and take it along with you wherever you go. Don't let it be the dictator of your life. You take control."

## JENNIFER ROBERGE:
## Trust Your Instincts and Keep Looking for Solutions

Jennifer Roberge was propelled to find solutions to her son's struggles with eczema, allergies, and asthma. She has since established herself as the go-to resource on integrative and holistic methods of healing eczema. Roberge is the founder of The Eczema Company, which features natural skin care, protective clothing, and other alternative products. She also created the award-winning blog *It's an Itchy Little World*. Roberge shared her story of her struggle to help her son with eczema during a phone interview for this book.

When Roberge's son was just a few months old, he developed red, dry, itchy patches of skin. Before long her baby was covered in eczema that looked like burns. She began using a number of creams and ointments prescribed by doctors and dermatologists, including topical corticosteroids. But no matter how diligently she applied these creams and ointments, her son's eczema kept coming back, and eventually the topical steroids seemed to stop working. Her son's doctors started prescribing stronger and stronger topical steroids, and Roberge grew more dismayed at watching her son suffer and not being able to help him.

At some point, her maternal-instinct alarm bells started going off. "It just didn't seem right. We were using stronger and stronger creams and he was just a child. It just seemed crazy. I kept wondering, is this going to go on forever?" Roberge says.

After taking a mandatory two-week break from topical steroids caused her son's skin to flare uncontrollably, she decided it was time for a change. As she lost faith in conventional methods of treating eczema, she began researching alternative methods and treatments. But at that time, around 2010, there wasn't a lot of information available about alternative or natural ways to manage eczema. She and her husband were also at odds over how to deal with their son's eczema. Her husband believed they should stick with conventional methods, but Roberge felt they needed to explore other options. The stress of it all took an enormous emotional toll on her and put a strain on her marriage.

"I was in my darkest time. I was searching the internet and hysterically crying and looking for solutions," Roberge says. "At one point I bought something from the Czech Republic. It was very rare to find products with hemp at that time. I couldn't even read the ingredient list. I just knew there was hemp in it, and I was so desperate that I got it. It didn't help him. I thought, this is crazy, what am I doing?"

They did an elimination diet and discovered that removing certain foods helped clear his skin up. At the time, it felt like a miracle, but she cautions families to do elimination diets with care. Her son also went on to develop several food allergies, including what she describes as a "full-blown" dairy allergy that caused him to have an anaphylactic reaction.

She is grateful that those dark times are largely behind them. Over time, she found natural products that helped soothe her son's skin, and he has outgrown his severe food allergies. The process of figuring out what works was slow, painful, and expensive. Just trying to locate natural or holistic products could be difficult. Roberge also began to realize that she wasn't alone;

so many parents like her were on a similar quest, all looking for options that might help their child with eczema.

"That's why I started the store, to make a place for parents who are looking for different options to choose from," Roberge says. "There's no one miracle product. There's no one product that's going to work for everybody. The product that I find works really well for my son may work well for five other kids. But there's 10 other kids it won't work for."

There are no "miracle cures" for eczema, Roberge explains. It often comes down to finding the right combination of things that seem to work best for you, and this often takes a great deal of trial and error. Offering different options for natural products and nontoxic skin care through her online store is one way Roberge feels she can help others.

Roberge regularly attends eczema conferences, and she has noticed that things are slowly changing and that people within the eczema community are becoming more open-minded about trying natural and alternative treatments and products. "Now they are talking more about diet and they're talking more about topical steroid addiction," Roberge says. "They are acknowledging that some of these things I was worried about are true."

# PETER TAPAO:
## Stay Focused and Fit

After a childhood of dealing with severe eczema and food allergies, Peter Tapao found his calling in fitness and exercise and ultimately helping others find their inner strength. Tapao shared his story of how he refused to let eczema keep him from his goals of physical fitness during a phone interview for this book.

Like many people with chronic eczema, Tapao was diagnosed with the chronic skin condition as a baby. Doctors advised his mother to apply Vaseline and hydrocortisone cream and said that hopefully it would go away. But over time as Tapao grew, the symptoms worsened and new ones appeared that were even more baffling to his mother and doctors.

As a young child, Tapao's body seemed to react to a number of things, ranging from foods to things in his environment. It seemed that after he ate certain foods, he would experience distressing symptoms such as vomiting, diarrhea, tightening and itching in his throat, and horrible skin hives in addition to the eczematous rash that always seemed present on his skin. At the time, in the early 1980s, eczema and food allergies were still relatively uncommon, and no one else in Tapao's family had experienced anything like this before. Doctors told his mother they weren't convinced he was reacting to food, and his mother was uncertain about what to do to help him.

What Tapao was going through was a progression of symptoms known as the "atopic march," or allergic march (which we'll talk about in depth in the next chapter). Tapao's mother did the best she could to seek medical treatment and help him with his cascading symptoms, but she faced an uphill battle on a number of fronts. Not long before Tapao was born, his parents had immigrated from the Philippines to the US to begin a new life in Northern California's Bay Area, but five months before Tapao was born, his father died in an accident. His grieving mother raised Tapao by herself with the help of extended family, but she faced her own sorrow and uncertainty about how to navigate a new country and culture.

"It was pretty rough for her," Tapao says. "After my father passed away, my mother went through a great despair. She had the help of my father's family, who were here, but she had a hard time engaging with everything going on."

Tapao suspected from a young age that he was reacting to the foods he ate, but at that time, the doctors he saw said he simply had eczema and dismissed the possibility that he had food or environmental allergies, or that there was a connection between those conditions.

"I remember leaving a doctor's office as a child after the doctor told me that I didn't have food allergies," says Tapao. "I remember thinking that I thought the doctor had it wrong. But at that time, in the 1980s, the doctors I saw didn't seem to know a lot about food allergies." His mother, baffled by her son's symptoms and the doctor's insistence that he didn't have food allergies, sought out alternative practitioners to help, but ultimately to no avail.

Later, in his twenties, Tapao finally went through testing and it was determined that he was, indeed, allergic to many common foods, including peanuts, eggs, and dairy, although thankfully he never experienced life-threatening symptoms such as anaphylaxis.

As a child, Tapao also began to have severe reactions whenever he was around dogs or cats, and he developed severe hay fever, especially to grass and other things in his environment. At the time, it all amounted to misery for Tapao as his undiagnosed food and environmental allergies seemed to cause continual eczema flares. And even when his skin wasn't flaring, teachers were aghast at the scars left on his skin.

The condition left him feeling anxious and deeply depressed at times, likely made worse because he had trouble sleeping at night. Tapao coped by turning his focus to things that brought him joy and gave him purpose. He began to use exercise and sports as a way to channel his anxiety and release negative emotions. He played football and basketball, and he excelled in the Filipino martial art of Escrima or Arnis.

"There were times when I felt like I could barely move, like I could barely get off the couch," Tapao says. "But then my inner persona would come out, like my inner trainer-bootcamp-guy came out, and I'd make myself get up and get going."

Working out and staying physically fit became a way to tackle his fears and depression. His love of sports became his escape, but it also helped him grow mentally stronger and more resilient.

"There were times I felt so ashamed. But for whatever reasons, I always had an outgoing personality," Tapao says.

When your skin feels like an open wound, it may be hard to contemplate exercise or being active. But for Tapao, the love of being physically active helped him through his darkest times. He also discovered a passion for helping others feel empowered and find their own inner strength. "I feel that if you are broken, you can help other people who are broken, and together you can make each other strong," he says.

Tapao is now a strength and conditioning coach, a group exercise instructor, and a personal trainer at the fitness facilities on the Facebook campus in Fremont and at a gym in Oakland, California. He helps organize endurance events such as Spartan Races and Tough Mudder runs.

Tapao has also been able to find relief from his eczema by using Dupixent (dupilumab), which has been like a miracle drug, he says. It has controlled his eczema and allowed him to focus on other things, like being a husband and a dad to three small children.

"I know how ugly it can be to sit in your own despair. I have been there a few times," Tapao says. "You have to focus on your strength and your dreams. You can't stop living your life or allow eczema to dictate who you are."

CHAPTER 5

# THE LINK BETWEEN ECZEMA AND OTHER ALLERGIC DISEASES

Chances are, if you have eczema, you also have allergies. For many people, atopic, or allergic, conditions often run together in what has been termed the "atopic march," or allergic march. The allergic march can include food allergies; environmental allergies, such as allergic rhinitis (hay fever); and allergies to animal dander, dust mites, or mold. In this chapter, we'll look at how researchers are working to unravel the complexities of the connection between eczema and allergic conditions.

Researchers have found that infants with atopic dermatitis are more likely to go on to develop these allergic conditions throughout their childhood. In fact, studies have found that 80 percent of children with chronic eczema develop asthma and/or hay fever later on, according to Dr. Asriani M. Chiu, professor of pediatrics (allergy and immunology) and medicine and director of the Asthma and Allergy Clinic at the Children's Hospital of Wisconsin/Medical College of Wisconsin. Chiu was interviewed through email for this book.

It also appears that the world is quickly becoming a more allergic place for many of us. Allergic diseases of all kinds have been increasing in recent decades and now affect more than 20 percent of the population worldwide. It may be that changes in everything from our diet, lifestyle, and outdoor activity levels have influenced our propensity to be more allergic. And this propensity is increased for those who had eczema as a baby, explains Dr. Ruchi S. Gupta, professor of pediatrics and medicine at Northwestern Medicine and director of the Center for Food Allergy & Asthma Research within Northwestern University Feinberg School of Medicine's Institute for Public Health and Medicine. Gupta was interviewed over email and she also shared several online videos and lectures she has given on the topic of eczema and allergies and how these two are so closely linked.

In addition to the atopic march, studies have found that food allergies can cause eczema flare-ups in some people, especially those who are under the age of five, while airborne substances such as pollen or spores are more likely to cause eczema in older children and adults.

## ECZEMA AND ALLERGIES: WHAT'S THE CONNECTION?

The concept of the atopic march was developed to describe the progression of symptoms that seem linked starting from a young age. Understanding "how" and "why" the allergic march develops is a topic of ongoing research, and great strides have been made in recent years, with compelling theories that link the health of our skin barrier to how our immune system becomes sensitized to allergies.

However, before we get into these theories, keep in mind that the development of allergic diseases can vary from person to person, and this progression is influenced by both genetic and environmental factors. Some people may develop some of these conditions in an unrelated fashion—it isn't clear what causes them to develop allergic conditions. Some people may "grow out" of some of these conditions or see their severity lessen over time. But others will deal with these chronic conditions for their entire life.

A growing body of evidence suggests that, for many people, eczema and allergies are connected and there may be steps that can be taken early on to lessen their impact. In particular, new guidelines advise parents on introducing certain highly allergenic foods to children who are believed to be at high risk for developing food allergies. Feeding these allergenic foods to babies earlier in life has been found to diminish the likelihood that they will develop food allergies. Of course, parents should only do so after thorough discussion with their child's pediatrician, who will likely provide a referral to an allergist/immunologist.

The allergic march begins with eczema, followed by a cascade of other allergic conditions, such as asthma, allergic rhinitis (hay fever), and food allergies. Beyond eczema appearing first, the other conditions don't necessarily follow a specific order, and not everyone develops all of these conditions. However, research shows that you have a higher chance of developing at least one of these allergic conditions if you had atopic dermatitis as an infant, explains Gupta, who has more than 15 years of experience as a board-certified pediatrician and health researcher.

## UNDERSTANDING WHAT MAKES US SNEEZE, ITCH, AND SWELL

We get allergies when our immune system reacts to a substance in our environment called an allergen. This might be something seemingly innocuous, such as pollen, food, dust, or mold, but for some people, the proteins in this substance cause the immune system to go a little haywire. You can be allergic to something you eat, something you inhale into your lungs, something your skin touches, or something injected into your body. According to the Asthma and Allergy Foundation of America, allergic conditions constitute the most common health issue affecting children in the US. More than 8.8 million children have skin allergies and more than 6.1 million children have hay fever. Overall, more than 50 million Americans experience allergies annually.

When your body comes into contact with a substance it considers to be abnormal, your immune system produces a protein called an antibody. Most of the time this will cause a fairly mild reaction. If you have seasonal allergies, spring, summer, and fall may find you constantly sneezing, with an itchy, running nose and red, watery eyes. Environmental allergies and asthma also often occur together, and the same substances that trigger hay fever can also trigger asthma symptoms. In some people, skin or food allergies, as well as exercise, infections, or even stress can also cause asthma symptoms.

Some people can develop severe allergic reactions to certain things, such as foods, insect stings, medications, and latex. If you become hypersensitive to one of these allergens, your immune system essentially overreacts by releasing a flood of chemicals that can cause extreme and potentially life-threatening symptoms called anaphylaxis. People who have both asthma and a food allergy are at greater risk for anaphylaxis.

Like eczema, there is no cure for allergies, but you can learn to manage them. One common way to treat allergies is by using antihistamines, decongestants, or nasal sprays. It can also be helpful to try rinsing your nasal passages with a saline solution.

If over-the-counter options don't work, consult your doctor. Testing can be done to determine what, exactly, you're allergic to so you can avoid those triggers. For some people, allergy shots (allergen immunotherapy) are effective in helping to desensitize their immune system to certain allergens.

## THE PREVALENCE OF FOOD ALLERGIES

Because food allergies can be potentially dangerous or even life-threatening, many parents are particularly concerned about the connection between eczema and food allergies. And for good reason, explains Gupta: having eczema is the number one risk factor for developing food allergies. That doesn't mean that if you have eczema, you will automatically develop food allergies. But if you had eczema as a baby, you're at higher risk for developing food allergies later on. Also concerning to many is the growing prevalence of food allergies worldwide.

According to a number of surveys of pediatricians and family practitioners, schoolteachers, school nurses, and the general public, the prevalence of food allergies in children has been increasing over the past two decades. Between 1997 and 2008, the prevalence of peanut or tree nut allergy appears to have more than tripled in US children. And the Centers for Disease Control and Prevention (CDC) reports that the prevalence of food allergies in children increased by 50 percent between 1997 and 2011.

Understanding the growing prevalence of food allergies in children was the focus of a large-scale study headed by Gupta. Using a nationally representative survey of more than 38,000 children sampled in 2015 and 2016, the study found that about 8 percent of children (or about 5.6 million children) in the United States have a food allergy. Of those children with a food allergy,

42 percent reported having a severe reaction, and 40 percent reported being allergic to multiple foods.

The prevalence of adults with food allergies is also growing. Almost 1 in 10 adults in the US report having a food allergy; however, some adults may believe they have a food allergy when they may actually have another food-related condition.

The most common food allergens in the US are milk, eggs, tree nuts, peanuts, fish, shellfish, wheat, and soy. Gupta's study also identified sesame as a common food allergy.

In particular, peanut allergies are on the rise. In 1999 peanut allergies affected 0.4 percent of children and 0.7 percent of adults in the US. By 2010 the prevalence of peanut allergies among children had increased to about 2 percent. And those who are allergic to peanuts may have more severe reactions. According to the American Academy of Allergy, Asthma & Immunology, reactions to peanut made up approximately 45 percent of food-induced anaphylaxis cases.

However, it is important to note that overall fatalities to food allergies—including peanut allergy—remains low. While researchers note that peanut allergy is the leading cause of death related to food-induced anaphylaxis in the US, overall, very few people die of anaphylactic reactions. Studies have estimated that anaphylaxis from food allergies cause about 100 deaths annually in the US. Peanut allergy often becomes evident during infancy and preschool years. Up to 22 percent of people will eventually outgrow their peanut allergy; most people will continue to be allergic throughout their lives.

If you have eczema, you're at an exponentially higher risk of developing a food allergy than the general population. According to Chiu, about 30 percent of patients with eczema have a confirmed food allergy. And compared with children who don't have food allergies, children with a food allergy are two to four times as likely to have other allergic conditions, such as asthma or eczema.

## CAN YOU OUTGROW FOOD ALLERGIES?

Most parents are hopeful that their child will outgrow a food allergy over time. This question was central to a large-scale study conducted by Gupta and her colleagues between June 2009 and February 2010, in which the families of 40,104 children nationwide were surveyed. The researchers analyzed data for nine common food allergies: milk, peanut, shellfish, tree nuts, egg, fin fish, wheat, soy, and sesame.

The study, published in 2013 in *Annals of Allergy, Asthma & Immunology*, found that 3,188 children surveyed currently had a food allergy, while 1,245 had outgrown one. Here are some of the study's key findings:

- More than a quarter of the children—26.6 percent— outgrew their allergies, at an average age of 5.4 years old.
- Children who were allergic to milk, egg, or soy were most likely to outgrow their allergies. The likelihood of outgrowing shellfish, tree nut, or peanut allergies was significantly lower.
- The earlier a child's first reaction, the more likely that child was to outgrow the allergy.

Other factors that correlated with outgrowing an allergy included having a history of only mild to moderate reactions, being allergic to only one food, and having eczema as the only symptom. Conversely, children with severe symptoms (trouble breathing, swelling, and anaphylaxis) and multiple food allergies were less likely to see their food allergies fade over time.

# WHY ARE WE BECOMING MORE ALLERGIC?

One theory about what's behind this increase in food and other allergies has been proposed by Professor Katie Allen, pediatric gastroenterologist and allergist at the Royal Children's Hospital in Melbourne, Australia. Allen summarizes her theory as "the five D's" (dry skin, diet, vitamin D, dogs, and dribble). In a nutshell, increasing allergies may be caused by these five factors:

- **Dry skin and diet**—having eczema as a baby (and thus having dry, cracked skin) puts you at higher risk for developing allergic conditions. Also, delaying giving babies allergenic foods could be doing more harm than good.

- **Vitamin D hypothesis**—are we getting too little vitamin D, and is this causing us to be more inclined to develop allergic conditions? Researchers have found that infants who are vitamin D deficient are 3 times more likely to have an egg allergy and 11 times more likely to have a peanut allergy.

- **Dogs and dribble**—or the hygiene hypothesis. Overall, we have become very clean; we use antibacterial soaps and avoid exposure to dirt and bacteria, but this may be causing some of our hypersensitivities to allergens. Some studies have found that having a dog in the house may help decrease the chances of developing allergies. It's also been found that living with an older sibling (and thus being exposed to another person's "dribble" and their microbiome) reduces a child's chances of developing allergies. Another study found that when babies used pacifiers that had been dropped on the ground, their risk of allergy was lower.

Overall, the idea is that getting kids outside more often and exposing them earlier on to allergenic foods, as well as to a mix of different bacteria and microbiomes, will make their immune systems more robust and less apt to be sensitized to allergens.

## THE DUAL-ALLERGEN HYPOTHESIS

As we discussed earlier, the skin functions as a barrier between the body and the outside world, keeping allergens, infections, and irritants out. People with eczema may have a skin barrier dysfunction that results in their skin becoming extremely dry, cracked, and inflamed. This broken skin may act as a kind of gateway, allowing allergens into the body in an abnormal way.

One groundbreaking hypothesis that examined this interplay between the skin barrier and the immune system is the dual-allergen hypothesis, first proposed by Dr. Gideon Lack, a pediatric allergist and researcher in the United Kingdom. Lack noticed that the rate of peanut allergy was 10 times higher among Jewish children in the UK than Israeli children. This huge discrepancy couldn't be explained by genetics, socioeconomics, or a tendency to develop other allergies. There was one major cultural difference between these two communities. In Israel, babies start eating foods containing peanuts when they are about seven months old, and they continue to eat peanut products as part of their regular diet. But in the UK, children usually don't consume any peanuts until they are a year old.

This led Lack to speculate that earlier consumption of peanut products might help protect against peanut allergy. What followed was the Learning Early About Peanut Allergy (LEAP) study, which was published in 2015 and showed that feeding peanut products to high-risk infants starting from about four months old and continuing to about five years old led to an 86 percent reduction in prevalence of peanut allergy.

LEAP compared two strategies to prevent peanut allergy: early consumption versus dietary avoidance of peanuts in babies who were at high risk for developing peanut allergy because they already had severe eczema, an egg allergy, or both. The study also excluded infants showing early strong signs of having already developed peanut allergy.

The hypothesis postulates that infants with eczema can be exposed to peanut proteins through their broken, rashy skin; this is called cutaneous exposure. If babies are exposed to these allergens before they eat them, they can have early sensitization to these proteins, which causes them to have a food allergy. In a National Eczema Association (NEA) webinar entitled "What about the Food? How Food Can Help or Harm Our Eczema." Gupta explains, "As an infant, if you're exposed cutaneously to some of the top allergens, such as peanut, dust, milk protein, egg protein—it has to be the protein because that's what our bodies are reacting to—this may skew their immune system and cause food allergies."

However, if infants are first exposed to the allergenic proteins orally, by eating and digesting the food in their guts, their immune systems are processing the allergen the "normal" way, and the child has a higher likelihood of being tolerant to the food, notes Gupta.

This study and a number of subsequent studies have gone a long way in explaining the relationship between eczema and food allergies and why having eczema, especially severe eczema, can be such a big risk factor for developing food allergies.

# NEW GUIDELINES FOR INTRODUCING ALLERGENIC FOODS

Prior to 2000, the American Academy of Pediatrics (AAP) suggested that introduction of certain highly allergenic foods be delayed in high-risk children. They said cow's milk should not be introduced until age one; eggs until age two; and peanuts, tree nuts, and fish until age three. But these new studies suggested that this delay was likely doing more harm than good.

Starting in 2017, new guidelines were put forward for when to introduce highly allergenic foods to babies—especially to those children considered to be at high risk of developing a food allergy. The AAP now supports the policy of early peanut introduction to high-risk babies and young children. However, if your child is at high risk for developing a food allergy, early peanut introduction should only be done after consulting your child's physician and possibly after allergy testing, Gupta says.

Pediatricians need to assess infants for severe to moderate eczema at their four-month well-child visit, Gupta explains in the NEA webinar. "If the infant has severe eczema, that infant needs to be managed," she explains. "That means giving them treatment for the eczema, but also the pediatrician needs to assess if the child has a specific IgE [a type of antibody] to peanut." If the test comes back positive for an IgE-mediated peanut allergy, then the baby should be referred to an allergist, recommends Gupta.

If the infant has moderate or even mild eczema, he or she should start being fed peanut products at home as soon as possible, around the age of six months, Gupta notes. Children may be introduced to peanuts that have been ground up or given in "puff" form, but never give a baby or young child whole peanuts, which are a choking hazard.

## FOOD-EXACERBATED ECZEMA

While eczema and food allergies are clearly linked, the subject of food allergens exacerbating or triggering an eczema flare-up has long been debated, studied, and discussed. Research shows that those most likely to be impacted by food-exacerbated eczema are infants and children with moderate to severe chronic eczema. The number of eczema patients whose skin symptoms are linked to food allergens varies depending on what study you're looking at. But anecdotally speaking, doctors note that many people with chronic eczema believe their skin condition is affected by what they eat.

It's important to listen to your body and note how it's reacting to the foods you eat. Research has found that dietary factors can indeed exacerbate atopic dermatitis or cause systemic contact dermatitis. Systemic contact dermatitis is a distinct T cell–mediated immunological reaction in which dietary exposure to specific allergens results in dermatitis. "Ingestion of a specific food can acutely cause a flare of a patient's eczema; this is a real thing," Gupta says in the NEA webinar. "A flare can occur in hours or days after eating something."

Studies have found that food can be the cause of worsening eczema in up to 33 percent of patients with severe eczema, in 10 to 20 percent of patients with moderate eczema, and in only 6 percent of patients with mild eczema, Gupta explains.

However, if your child's eczema improves while eating an unrestricted diet, it's unlikely that food is triggering eczema flare-ups. If you think that food may be a trigger, it's important to see an allergy specialist and have an evaluation, Gupta says. It's also important to avoid unnecessarily limiting your child's diet; as we've seen from the LEAP study, avoiding a potential allergen may lead to the development of food allergies.

## WHAT IS A "TRUE" FOOD ALLERGY?

Many people are unaware that there is a significant difference between having a food allergy and having a food sensitivity or intolerance.

A true food allergy begins with your immune system. The immune system works by detecting and destroying harmful things in our bodies that make us sick, such as bacteria or viruses. In people with food allergies, the immune system is triggered to attack a food protein. When the body detects an offending food protein, it responds by making its own proteins, called immunoglobulin E (IgE) antibodies, to fight against that specific food allergen. These IgE molecules then attach themselves to mast cells, a type of white blood cell that produces histamine and other immune system substances.

The first time this happens to you, your body becomes "sensitized" to the food allergen, so that when you eat or drink that food again, the IgE antibodies detect it and signal the mast cells to release histamine and other inflammatory chemicals to attack the allergen. This process causes an allergic reaction, which can vary in severity.

# FOOD ALLERGY SYMPTOMS

While you can be allergic to any food, there are certain foods that tend to be more allergenic than others. Under the Food Allergen Labeling and Consumer Protection Act, the most common allergenic foods—which account for roughly 90 percent of food allergies—must be labeled. Often referred to as the "Big Eight," they are milk, eggs, peanuts, tree nuts (including almonds, walnuts, pecans, and cashews), fish, shellfish, soy, and wheat.

Food allergies can affect any system within the body. Here are some common major body symptoms:

- **Lower respiratory**—coughing, wheezing, trouble breathing
- **Upper respiratory**—runny nose, congestion, sneezing
- **Skin:** rashes, hives, swelling, itching (eczema flare-up)
- **Cardiovascular**—immediate drop in blood pressure, fainting, shortness of breath
- **Oral**—tingling, itching in the mouth, swelling in the mouth, trouble swallowing, feeling like your throat is closing

Other general symptoms of food allergies can include dizziness and lightheadedness, turning blue, and feeling confused or weak. Even trace amounts of a food allergen can cause a reaction. Some people may even have reactions from inhaling a food protein (such as in steam) or just touching the food.

According to the organization Food Allergy Research and Education (FARE), a child might describe a food allergy reaction by saying things like the following:

- "My tongue is hot (or burning)."

- "My tongue feels like there's hair on it."
- "My mouth is tingling (or feels itchy)."
- "My mouth feels funny."
- "It feels like a bump is on the back of my tongue."
- "There's something stuck in my throat."
- "My throat feels thick."
- "My lips feel tight."
- "It feels like there are bugs inside my ear."

Severe symptoms, either alone or combined with milder symptoms, may be signs of life-threatening anaphylaxis, or a serious allergic reaction. Prompt treatment is required, with epinephrine (a medication that constricts blood vessels and opens the airways in the lungs) being the first-line treatment. Once a serious allergic reaction begins, epinephrine is the only effective treatment to reduce your body's allergic response.

# FOOD ALLERGIES VS. FOOD INTOLERANCE

If your symptoms only seem to involve one system in the body, it may be that you have a food intolerance, sensitivity, or another type of food allergy. Each of these issues has different levels of severity and may be treated a little differently, Gupta explains. However, food intolerances or sensitivities don't involve the immune system, and they generally aren't as dangerous because there isn't a risk of having an anaphylactic reaction.

There are various reasons for food intolerances. For instance, your body might not produce the right enzymes to digest a certain food, or you might be sensitive to certain sugars or to chemicals like caffeine. One of the most common intolerances is lactose intolerance, which is when the body lacks the proper enzyme to break down the sugar in milk and dairy products.

# OTHER TYPES OF FOOD ALLERGIES

There is also a subset of food allergies that, while not usually life-threatening, can cause a person to become very ill. These are called non-IgE-mediated food allergies, which are caused by a reaction involving other components of the immune system apart from IgE antibodies. The symptoms of non-IgE reactions are usually delayed, and they usually affect the digestive tract, with symptoms such as vomiting, diarrhea, or bloating. There are no blood or skin tests to accurately determine if you have this type of allergy, so diagnosis must be made based on your history and whether your symptoms improve when the suspected food is removed from your diet.

Food protein–induced enterocolitis syndrome (FPIES) is an uncommon type of non-IgE-mediated food allergy that is usually seen in babies. It can cause profuse vomiting two to four hours after ingestion of a food, such as cow's milk or soy milk. It usually occurs soon after the food is introduced into the infant's diet. The reaction can be severe.

Eosinophilic esophagitis (EoE) is another non-IgE-mediated food allergy; it is more common in patients who have other allergic conditions, such as eczema. This allergy is characterized by difficulty swallowing, vomiting, and failure to thrive. Some studies have found that the development of EoE can be a late step in the progression of the atopic march. Babies who have eczema, food allergies, and asthma are at the highest risk for developing EoE.

Oral allergy syndrome (OAS), also known as pollen-food syndrome, is caused by a cross-reaction to food and pollen allergens in patients who are allergic to pollen. The most common symptom of this allergy is that when you eat a certain food, your mouth and palate immediately begin itching and tingling. This usually goes away after the food is swallowed or removed from the mouth. OAS typically presents in older children, teens, and young adults, and most people are only affected by raw fruits or vegetables—they can usually eat these same foods if they have been cooked. If you have seasonal allergies to pollen, you could potentially have these symptoms.

# ALLERGY ANTIBODY TESTING

If you're dealing with eczema and suspected food allergies, you may have had lab work for allergy testing done. One common allergy test looks at your immunoglobulin E (IgE) levels. IgE is an allergy antibody, specifically an immune protein, that is associated with allergic reactions. It is normally found in small amounts in the blood, but if you have a predisposition to allergies and are exposed to a potential allergen (such as a particular food, grass, or animal dander), your body may perceive the potential allergen as a foreign substance and react by producing a specific IgE antibody. If you suspect you are allergic to something specific, a blood test can be done to check the level of IgE antibodies specific to that allergen, says Chiu.

However, allergy testing doesn't always show the complete picture, and its results are often inconclusive. Because of this, Chiu does not recommend routine allergy testing for all patients with eczema, unless a patient or their family has noticed symptoms related to food that seem to be reproducible (for instance, if every time your child consumes milk or eggs, they always have specific symptoms).

Sometimes a patient or their family notices that a specific food seems to be causing a rash. In this case, the allergy specialist may still decide that it is not necessary to do testing, Chiu explains. The patient can do a two-week trial of avoidance to the specific food to see if that helps the skin. If it doesn't help, the food can be reintroduced. A food avoidance test can be informative to the allergist in determining if a food is worsening symptoms such as eczema.

## FOOD CHALLENGE TEST

The gold standard for testing and determining whether you have a food allergy is doing a food challenge test. Because this test can cause serious allergic reactions, including anaphylaxis, it should be conducted by an experienced allergist at a medical facility. During the challenge, the allergist feeds you the allergenic food in small, measured doses that are unlikely to trigger symptoms. You will wait for a period of time between each dose to see if you have a reaction.

If you continue to have no significant symptoms, you will gradually receive larger and larger doses. If you show signs of a reaction, the food challenge is stopped. If you have no symptoms by the end of the procedure, it's safe to rule out a food allergy. If the test confirms the food allergy, you will receive guidance on avoiding that particular food and you may be prescribed medications, such as an epinephrine autoinjector (EpiPen), which allows you to self-administer an epinephrine injection if you accidentally ingest the food and experience a life-threatening reaction.

# ALLERGY SKIN TEST

Another test you can do is an allergy skin test, which is also done in a doctor's office. A medical professional will expose your skin to a suspected allergen and then observe to see if there's a reaction. Allergy skin tests can help diagnose allergic conditions such as hay fever, allergic asthma, eczema, food allergies, penicillin allergy, bee venom allergy, or latex allergy.

The benefit of a skin test is that it gives fast results—usually within 20 minutes to a few hours—so you don't need to wait weeks to get the results, as you do with an allergy antibody test. A skin test also usually costs less than allergy blood tests. However, be aware that the state of your skin can make a difference; it can be hard to get a definitive reading if you're having an eczema flare-up. Also, certain medicines may interfere with the accuracy of the test, and the skill of the tester can also affect the results.

There are two types of skin tests. During a skin prick test, a drop of suspected allergen is pricked on the surface of the skin, usually on the back or the forearm. A number of suspected allergens can be tested at the same time. If you are allergic to one of these allergens, that test spot will become red and swollen.

The second type is called an intradermal skin test. It involves taking a small amount of a suspected allergen and injecting it into the skin of the arm. Like the skin prick test, a number of allergens can be tested at the same time.

# ASSESSING THE SEVERITY OF YOUR CHILD'S ECZEMA

Keep in mind that one of the most crucial ways to potentially prevent some of these allergies is to aggressively manage a baby's eczema early on. In fact, maintaining the skin is likely the most important way to mitigate eczema and potentially other allergies, so this is what Chiu and Gupta say they focus on first. This is where parents are key in providing the necessary support and being their child's best advocate in ensuring they're getting the proper treatment for their skin. "It's important to make sure to keep the skin hydrated by bathing daily, using moisturizers/ emollients, and using products that are nonirritating, like fragrance and dye-free cleansers, lotions, and detergents," Chiu notes.

This also means that pediatricians are at the forefront in diagnosing and treating eczema and are also the ones who will assess the severity of eczema cases. Gupta advises parents that if their child has eczema, it's important to ask the child's pediatrician how he or she assesses and manages eczema.

Assessing the severity of a child's eczema isn't always straightforward, explains Gupta. There are several tools that doctors can use to determine the severity of eczema, although these tools were primarily designed for use in clinical trials, and not necessarily for regular office visits with patients.

One such assessment tool is the SCORAD (scoring atopic dermatitis) system, which takes into account three main factors:

- **Body surface area**—To what extent does eczema cover a patient's skin?

- **Intensity**—This is determined by looking at different areas that demonstrate how intense the eczema is presenting on the skin, including redness, swelling, oozing/crusting, scratch marks, dryness, and skin thickening or lichenification, which is when skin develops thick, leathery patches. Each of these areas can be rated none, mild, moderate, or severe.

- **Subjective symptoms**—This is the patient's recollection of itchiness (pruritus), or the urge to scratch, and sleeplessness.

Using the SCORAD system, a doctor will take all of these areas into account to compile a score and determine how severe a patient's eczema is. However, this may not be practical for a pediatrician to do with a young child.

A simpler tool is the Validated Investigator Global Assessment scale for Atopic Dermatitis (vIGA-AD scale), which rates severity from 0 to 4, with 0 being no signs of eczema and 4 being severe eczema (widespread across the body and with deep or bright red skin, along with swelling or thickening of the skin). Parents should be aware that these scales are subjective to the physician or the pediatrician using the tools to assess their patients, Gupta explains. Gupta discusses this in a PeerView Institute video "A Closer Look at the Atopic Dermatitis Patient Journey: Effective Management Approaches Across the Age and Disease Spectrum." PeerView Institute provides continuing education and professional development to physicians and other healthcare professionals.

"As pediatricians, we're on the front lines to assess atopic dermatitis in infants," Gupta explains in the video. "It is our job to manage it appropriately and to refer them as needed to the dermatologist or allergists, so that they can protect that skin barrier as early as possible to potentially prevent other comorbidities."

# CAN BREASTFEEDING HELP PREVENT THE ATOPIC MARCH?

While there is a great deal of interest in finding ways to prevent eczema and allergies from developing, we still don't have definitive answers, notes Chiu. Besides the recommendation to introduce allergenic foods earlier, the AAP also recommends exclusively breastfeeding for its potential protective benefits against eczema.

Although the data on the benefits of breastfeeding and eczema is still limited and some data is conflicting, studies have linked breastfeeding with decreased food allergies and eczema. One study found that a mother's diet may help protect her newborn against developing food allergies later on. Other studies have found that breastfeeding can promote tolerance to foods that most often cause allergies. And some data suggests that breastfeeding may decrease the incidence of eczema during the first two years of life and may also be protective against wheezing or developing asthma even after five years of age. Exclusively breastfeeding for at least three months was also associated with a significantly lower chance of continued eczema flare-ups when a child was six years old. Although breastfeeding may not prevent eczema altogether, it has played a protective role in decreasing the chronic nature of the skin disease into childhood.

"We strongly recommend breast feeding, if possible, for the first 6 to 12 months," explains Chiu in an email interview. Then parents can move on to solid foods in stage-appropriate forms when the child is ready, including introducing allergenic foods sooner rather than later, Chiu adds.

# CHAPTER 6

# HOLISTIC AND ALTERNATIVE TREATMENT OPTIONS

Tormented by eczema her whole life, Rebecca Bonneteau was in her early thirties when she made the radical decision to leave her corporate job as a business analyst and go back to school to study alternative medicine in a quest to heal herself from the inside out. While conventional medicine wanted to treat her chronic eczema as a problem unto itself, with treatments focused on managing and controlling symptoms on the skin, she believed that there must be more to it. She felt certain her lifelong skin problems were part of an underlying, internal issue, and she was determined to fix it.

Bonneteau, who lives in the United Kingdom, spent four years studying to become a naturopath, nutritionist, and iridologist (iridology is an alternative medicine technique of examining the irises for information on a patient's systemic health). Now, more than six years after she started this journey, Bonneteau says that not only is her eczema mostly gone but she is also using her knowledge to help others tackle the root problems underlying their eczema. Bonneteau has branded herself as "The Eczema Expert." She takes on patients from across the globe, consulting with them via video chat and recommending a variety of natural treatments, including essential oils, herbs, herbal teas, tinctures, and dietary changes. Bonneteau was interviewed for this book over video chat.

Bonneteau and her patients are among a growing trend of people seeking alternative forms of treatment, in part because they are discouraged and fed up with conventional treatments. This exasperation and frustration among eczema patients is something Dr. Peter Lio often sees in his role as clinical assistant professor of dermatology and pediatrics at Northwestern University Feinberg School of Medicine and in his private practice at Medical Dermatology Associates of Chicago.

Alternative medicine generally isn't evidence-based and doesn't have robust clinical studies to back up treatments—a mainstay in conventional medicine. Yet more people are turning to alternative medicine than ever before. For Lio, the answer to the question of how to best bridge this gap between conventional and alternative is to embrace both and offer patients options from both. This is his goal as founding director of the Chicago Integrative Eczema Center.

Lio hopes that patients can reap the benefits of both prudent conventional medical knowledge and the more holistic, mind-spirit-body approach of alternative medicine.

## A GROWING TREND TOWARD ALTERNATIVE AND NATURAL THERAPIES

Complementary and alternative medicine (CAM) have been growing in popularity, and people are increasingly becoming interested in using these treatments to address all manner of chronic ailments and diseases. According to a survey by the National Center for Complementary and Integrative Health (a US government agency), nearly 40 percent of adults and about 12 percent of children in the US use some form of complementary and alternative medicine.

In the world of dermatology, studies have found that more than 50 percent of eczema patients have tried one or more forms of alternative medicine, as Lio reports in a 2011 *Practical Dermatology* article. Unsurprisingly, this growing interest in alternative medicine coincides with a deepening frustration with conventional methods, especially when they aren't able to effectively treat poorly understood chronic conditions like eczema.

When it comes to the dermatological issues, Lio believes that patients turn to alternative medicine for several reasons:

- Dealing with a disease like eczema that is incurable
- Feeling unsatisfied with their doctor's explanations and lack of answers for this disease
- Being given treatments that have a perceived safety risk or prescribed treatments that only treat symptoms but don't address deeper issues

Conventional medical knowledge still comes up short when you're dealing with a chronic and incurable disease like eczema, acknowledges Lio. Doctors still don't fully understand how the disease develops, so people are left feeling frustrated by a lack of information and treatment options. In addition, people don't always connect with their physicians, and they may feel like they aren't being heard or their needs aren't being met. This can make alternative options more appealing.

# WHAT IS ALTERNATIVE MEDICINE?

Alternative medicine encompasses a huge range of practices, theories, modalities, treatments, and products that are believed to have healing effects but that aren't generally used in standard medicine and aren't based on established scientific methods. If you use an alternative treatment in conjunction with conventional medical treatments, it's referred to as a complementary treatment. So complementary and alternative medicine is the umbrella term that can encompass anything that doesn't fit into the neat box of conventional medicine.

CAM can be broken up into several broad categories. These can include traditional or alternative medical systems that were developed apart from conventional or Western medical practices. Some traditional medical systems are thousands of years old and based on ancient philosophies and methodologies. Some alternative medical systems are much newer.

In addition to alternative or traditional medical modalities, there are a number of alternative treatments or natural remedies, which are also included under the broad category of CAM. These can include natural approaches or using substances found in nature for medicinal or therapeutic purposes. Specific natural remedies and approaches are discussed further in Chapter 8.

Many forms of alternative medicine take a holistic approach, which means that they consider the person as a whole and look at the deeper connections between body, mind, and spirit. The principles behind holistic medicine include the following:

• Each person has innate healing powers.

• Each person has a unique makeup, so most treatments need to be individualized.

• Treating a condition involves fixing the underlying cause, not just alleviating symptoms.

# INTEGRATIVE MEDICINE

Some conventional physicians, such as Lio, believe that the best outcomes happen when alternative medicine is integrated with conventional approaches. This is called integrative medicine, and it combines conventional medical practices with alternative medical practices that have been shown to have some high-quality scientific evidence of safety and effectiveness. These integrative practices can include things like acupuncture, yoga, or massage and often focus on the patient's nutrition and health habits.

Lio, who is also an acupuncturist, says he favors this blended, integrative approach because it offers patients the best of both worlds. And the trend appears to be picking up steam in the conventional medical world. In fact, the American Board of Physician Specialties (ABPS) even offers board certification in integrative medicine. According to the ABPS, physicians with this certification are "committed to a practice of medicine that reaffirms the relationship between practitioner and patient, focuses on the whole person, is informed by evidence, and makes use of all appropriate therapeutic approaches and disciplines to achieve optimal health and healing."

# HOLISTIC HEALTH PRACTITIONERS

Many people turn to holistic health practitioners or natural healers to help treat chronic conditions such as eczema. These practitioners use different alternative medicine and holistic health modalities to inform their practice and the approaches they take in treating patients. There are a myriad of alternative or holistic modalities out there, but in general, holistic practitioners focus on treating the "whole person" and not just alleviating a set of symptoms. From the holistic viewpoint, most diseases are a symptom of something deeper that has gone awry, so "fixing" the problem means correcting the underlying issue. This is why many holistic practitioners believe that eczema is more than skin deep and that a lasting solution requires that the patient explore what is happening internally.

The way Bonneteau explains it, the big difference between conventional methods and a natural or holistic approach to treating eczema is that a holistic approach focuses on healing eczema from the inside out. That means identifying the underlying issues in your body's systems that are ultimately triggering eczema flares. A holistic treatment plan usually involves weaving together healing practices for the mind, body, and spirit, says Tara Cameron, who is a licensed acupuncturist and East Asian medicine practitioner specializing in nutrition and herbal medicine. Cameron herself has dealt with chronic eczema and has experienced a condition called topical steroid withdrawal as a result of using topical steroids to control flare-ups. She also runs an online support group for people with eczema who are going through topical steroid withdrawal. Cameron was interviewed by phone for this book.

Some practitioners, including Cameron, study multiple holistic modalities so that they can use various holistic approaches or techniques when dealing with patients. Cameron likens this to having multiple tools in her toolbox to help her meet patients where they're at and give them the support they need. But because alternative therapies work differently for each person, it may take some time to see which holistic treatments work best for you.

# ALTERNATIVE MEDICINE APPROACHES FOR ECZEMA

Alternative medicine approaches that are commonly used for eczema include naturopathy, homeopathy, Ayurveda, Traditional Chinese Medicine, and functional medicine.

## Naturopathy

Naturopathy, or naturopathic medicine, aims to help the body heal through natural substances such as food and herbs. The American Association of Naturopathic Physicians defines naturopathic medicine as "emphasizing prevention, treatment, and optimal health through the use of therapeutic methods and substances that encourage individuals' inherent self-healing process. The practice of naturopathic medicine includes modern and traditional, scientific, and empirical methods."

When treating eczema, a naturopathic practitioner will look to identify and treat underlying causes that can contribute to eczema. Naturopathic practitioners may recommend herbal salves and creams or tinctures that are taken internally. They may also recommend dietary changes to include more nutrient-dense, clean foods as well as nutritional supplements or the use of probiotics, and they may recommend removing foods from the diet that cause inflammation. They will look to minimize your exposure to toxins and also provide mental and emotional stress support.

Some common botanical ingredients that may be used by naturopaths include calendula, lavender, chamomile, rose, Manuka honey, and tea tree, among many others.

# Homeopathy

This method is based on the belief that the body can cure itself. According to the British Homeopathic Association, homeopathy is based on the principle of "like cures like." In other words, a substance taken in extremely small amounts will cure the same symptoms it causes if taken in large amounts. Homeopathic medicines—known as "remedies"—are made from tiny amounts of certain natural substances, such as plants and minerals, to treat various ailments.

Homeopaths believe that the lower the dose, the more powerful the medicine. In fact, many of these remedies no longer contain any molecules of the original substance. Homeopathic remedies come in a variety of forms, such as sugar pellets, liquid drops, creams, gels, and tablets. Examples of remedies that may be used to treat eczema include sulfur, calcarea carbonica, and arsenicum album. Lio notes that while some eczema patients swear by homeopathy, the data from studies shows that homeopathic remedies don't work in a consistent or reliable way.

# Ayurveda

Ayurvedic medicine is a system of natural healing that has its origins in the Vedic culture of India. It is based on the belief that your health and wellness depend on a delicate balance between the mind, body, and spirit. According to the National Ayurvedic Medical Association (NAMA), "with a unique emphasis on total wellness, the art and science of Ayurveda work to harmonize our internal and external worlds."

Ayurveda is based on "the five great elements": ether, air, fire, water, and earth. As NAMA explains on its website, "our five senses serve as the portals between the internal and external realms," as the five elements "dance the dance of creation around and within us." Ayurveda focuses on improving overall health and balance based on your own unique body constitution. According to Ayurveda, eczema is caused by diet and lifestyle, which leads to impaired digestion and the accumulation of toxins in the body's tissues.

In treating eczema, Ayurveda aims to improve the skin by improving the immune system of a person, which is achieved by removing these toxins and even controlling the mind. The goal is to purify the body and boost the immune system and generally "cool the fire" that has caused the imbalance in your body.

Ayurvedic treatment is individualized and includes specialized herbal combinations and diet. General advice on diet and lifestyle could include avoiding spicy or oily foods, tea, coffee, or hot spices as well as hot, humid environments.

## Traditional Chinese Medicine

This healing approach originated in China and has evolved over thousands of years. It is widely practiced in a number of countries as part of mainstream medicine. Traditional Chinese Medicine (TCM) is based on the theory that all the body's organs support each other, so all of our bodily systems and functions must be in balance. Treatments are intended to promote self-healing and are customized for the individual person.

Some Western-trained physicians are conducting research and clinical trials on how TCM can be used more widely within mainstream medicine, particularly in the treatment of eczema. Dr. Xiu-Min Li, a professor of pediatrics in the Division of Pediatric Allergy and Immunology at the Icahn School of Medicine at Mount Sinai in New York, is among a group of doctors who have been researching how TCM and Chinese herbal medicines can be especially helpful for those who are dealing with severe allergies, food allergies, and asthma.

TCM includes a number of component practices. Some of these practices, such as acupuncture, have become mainstream and have been incorporated into Western medical practices. Many of these practices are being used in the treatment of eczema. They can include the following:

- **Acupuncture**—This practice involves inserting very thin needles lightly into the patient's skin. This stimulates acupressure points, releasing qi (vital energy that flows through the body). Western doctors believe that acupuncture stimulates endorphins, natural chemicals in the body that block pain signals. Alternatively, manual pressure can also be used on acupressure points. Acupuncture has been studied for its benefits for many types of pain, and it can help control the itchiness and inflammation associated with eczema. Reducing itchiness is key to breaking the itch-scratch cycle that drives inflammation and redness.

- **Cupping therapy**—Long used in Traditional Chinese Medicine and other ancient healing systems, cupping has increased in popularity in recent years. This practice involves creating suction on the skin by placing rounded inverted cups onto certain parts of the body. It is believed that this helps increase blood flow to that area, although it may leave bruises on a person's skin where blood vessels burst from the suction effects. Cupping is also linked to acupoints on a person's body, which are central to the practice of acupuncture and acupressure.

- **Moxibustion**—This is the burning of herbal leaves on or near the body, a form of fire heat treatment that is believed to stimulate specific acupuncture points of the body. This has been used as a complementary treatment for allergy relief and may be recommended to help treat eczema.

- **Chinese herbal medicine**—These remedies are mainly plant based, but some preparations include minerals or animal products. They can be packaged as powders, pastes, lotions, or tablets, depending on the herb and its intended use. Different herbs have different properties and can balance particular parts of the body. When prescribing a particular herb or concoction of herbs, a TCM practitioner must take into account the state of the patient's yin (the feminine, receptive principle in nature) and yang (the male, active principle in nature) and the elements that are governing the affected organs.

## Functional Medicine

This is considered a form of alternative medicine, but it takes some conventional medical practices and scientific knowledge and integrates them with nonconventional practices. It might sound similar to integrative medicine, but functional medicine is entirely different. While integrative medicine is built on the foundation of conventional medicine, its approach is focused on a personalized health-care philosophy that sees each person as genetically and biochemically unique. It believes in supporting the normal healing mechanism of the body naturally, rather than attacking the disease directly.

Functional medicine seeks to determine how and why illness occurs and then address those issues, not just symptoms of the disease. The functional medicine approach is highly personalized and often includes a detailed analysis of an individual's genetic makeup and predisposing factors such as family history, lifestyle, past illness, and exposures.

When it comes to treating eczema, a functional medicine practitioner will evaluate a patient's "antecedents, triggers, and mediators." This includes looking at issues such as a hormone imbalance, depleted nutrients, impaired liver function, and "leaky gut" (which we'll discuss further in Chapter 7). A functional medicine practitioner will likely examine a patient's diet to see if food may be triggering a response.

## MIND-BODY PRACTICES

Many people find that their bouts of eczema worsen when they're under stress. Some mind-body practices have proven helpful in dealing with stress because these practices can help a person better cope with physical pain and learn to release negative emotions such as feelings of anxiety. There are a number of techniques that fall into this category. Examples include acupuncture (which we discuss above), tai chi, massage therapy, meditation, mindfulness, yoga, hypnosis, and biofeedback.

These practices have all been used in varying ways to help people with eczema. Some people have found that mind-body practices help them relax, relieve stress and anxiety, and ultimately stop the itch-scratch cycle. Mind-body practices are usually considered complementary in that they are typically done in conjunction with other treatments, which may include conventional medical treatments or other alternative or holistic treatments. Below we'll look at a few of the mind-body practices that some people with eczema have found helpful.

**Hypnotherapy and Biofeedback**—Stress is known to play a role in eczema flares, and non-pharmacological treatments such as hypnotherapy and biofeedback may be helpful in enhancing relaxation. Lio notes that scratching eczema can become a behavioral and conditioned response, especially during times of stress or when a person is feeling anxious. Some studies have found that biofeedback and hypnotherapy have been effective in reducing the severity of eczema symptoms and promoting better sleep.

Hypnotherapy is the use of guided hypnosis, where a person is put into a trance-like state of focus and concentration with the help of a clinical hypnotherapist. In this state, the person can turn their attention inward to help them regain control of certain areas of their life. Hypnotherapy can help people to relax and to better cope with the itch-scratch cycle.

Biofeedback is a technique that involves using visual or auditory feedback to help you gain control over some of your body's functions, such as lowering heart rate, lowering blood pressure, and reducing stress. The goal of biofeedback is to make subtle changes to the body, such as relaxing certain muscles and slowing your breathing. There are different types of biofeedback, but all involve wearing electrical sensors or devices that measure physiological changes, such as your heart rate or skin changes.

**Meditation**—This can be a simple, natural, and inexpensive way to deal with stress and anxiety. Researchers have reported that meditation can be a viable way to help people cope during eczema flares. The National Eczema Society funded a study that found that consistent use of meditation helped people improve their concentration and gave them a sense of control over their itch. Most meditation practices are meant to help you focus on the present and gain a new perspective on a stressful situation, such as your itchy skin, and help you combat negative thoughts.

**Emotional Freedom Technique (EFT)**—This practice is known by several names, including tapping or psychological acupressure. Emotional freedom technique is believed to create a balance in your energy system and treat pain. EFT is based on principles similar to those of acupuncture or acupressure, focusing on meridian points or energy hot spots to restore balance to your body's energy.

It involves tapping specific points on the body, primarily on the head and the face, in a particular sequence. While doing this, the person focuses on the issue that they wish to treat. The method first came to prominence in the 1990s when its founder, Gary Craig, published information about the therapy on his website. Certain EFT practices have been developed for eczema and other skin problems, and some proponents say it helps itching subside.

## MEETING WITH A NATURAL HEALER

If you have gotten used to having relatively short appointments with a conventional doctor, you may be pleasantly surprised by the personal attention a holistic practitioner gives to patients. Most holistic practitioners offer expanded appointment times that are longer than you would typically get with a conventional physician. For instance, Cameron usually schedules 90-minute appointments with her patients, and Bonneteau regularly schedules hour or longer video time slots with her patients.

Cameron believes that this time is key to building a strong foundational relationship with her patients. This isn't a one-directional, rigid relationship such as you would get with a conventional physician, she says. Instead, Cameron focuses on connecting with her patients in a deeper way. She begins her treatments by spending time talking with the person, seeing how they're doing in their daily lives and what outside issues may be influencing or affecting them, as well going over any internal or bodily problems. Everything from the patient's relationships with their family to how they're doing with their diet and nutrition is part of the discussion, Cameron explains.

Based on what she learns through this dialogue, Cameron draws from various tools to offer her patient a treatment plan. This often includes a mind/body treatment such as acupuncture, which she uses to help balance out the patient's nervous system response. She will also do EFT tapping and work on breathing techniques with them.

## FEELING CONNECTED TO YOUR PRACTITIONER

Many people who seek out a holistic practitioner do so after feeling dissatisfied with the care they received from conventional physicians, both Bonneteau and Cameron note in their interviews. The patients they see often feel distraught over their experiences with medical professionals, and they don't know where to turn; many patients are at the point where they want to investigate treatments for themselves.

"By the time people see me, they are just burnt out on conventional doctors," Cameron says. "They don't feel that anyone is listening to them." With that in mind, Cameron focuses on meeting the patients where they're at emotionally, physically, and spiritually, and being able to support their needs in all of these realms.

The relationship you have with a holistic practitioner is likely going to be very different from one you have with a conventional doctor, notes Cameron. Whereas a conventional doctor is directing and dictating your care, often a holistic practitioner is experimenting to see what feels right to you. For instance, Cameron focuses on building a foundational "reciprocal relationship" with her patients, where both parties are learning from each other and are able to have an open discourse. Your practitioner is ultimately your advocate who is helping you determine what tools work best for you, Cameron says.

It's important that you resonate and feel comfortable with your practitioner. Cameron says that, early on, she tells her patients that she is committed to helping them do the work necessary to get better, but that they should give themselves permission to leave at any time if they so desire.

## WORKING THROUGH THE TRAUMA OF ECZEMA

Many holistic practitioners feel that it's important to offer support in a variety of ways to help their patients attain both emotional and physical health. You may find that a holistic practitioner acts as life-coach, counselor, mind/body therapist, and alternative medicine healer.

One area that isn't always obvious to people who are dealing with chronic eczema—or to those who are supporting them— is the amount of trauma and mental anguish connected to this condition, Cameron explains. Trauma linked to eczema is largely hidden from view—it's not nearly as visible as the physical inflammation and redness. A holistic practitioner is often more attuned to the mental and emotional pain you are dealing with along with your physical symptoms. True healing comes after processing the emotional trauma you have been through as well, Cameron explains.

This trauma can have a mental impact, which can also contribute to the physical part of this disease. The mind, spirit, and body are intertwined and connected, so you can't focus on treating the body without also offering support for the mind and spirit, Cameron says. Eczema can affect your life and your quality of life in a multitude of ways, and it's important to address all of these elements as part of your holistic treatment.

Many of Bonneteau's patients are young children who are dealing with chronic eczema. Sometimes it's not just the patient who is dealing with the emotional trauma, but also parents and caregivers who are grappling with their own anguish over watching their loved one wrestle with chronic eczema. Sometimes parents bear the brunt of these emotions—more than they realize, she says.

Bonneteau gives herself and her parents as an example. She says her mother will sometimes recall horrific memories of Bonneteau's childhood, when her eczema was flaring out of control. Her mother remembers walking into Bonneteau's room in the morning to find her daughter covered in blood from scratching all night. Bonneteau, who is now in her late thirties, doesn't remember these incidents; she was either too young or those memories have been lost to her. But her mother still carries the memories. Bonneteau says it's important for parents not to diminish their own emotions and to make time to process and work through these feelings.

# FOOD AND NUTRITION TO HEAL

Many holistic practitioners also study nutrition and may recommend certain diets, supplements, or herbal remedies as part of your treatment. There are a number of diets that nutritionists and alternative medicine practitioners believe can help heal eczema. These diets run the gamut. For instance, in some forms of traditional medicine, eczema is believed to be caused by excess fire in the body, so it's recommended to balance your diet by eating "cooling" foods and herbs. In TCM, such foods include watermelon, cucumber, broccoli, apples, citrus fruits, peppermint, and cilantro.

In addition to diets, many holistic and alternative practices include using a variety of nutritional supplements or herbs that are believed to help support the body and decrease eczema symptoms. We'll look at some of these specific diets and supplements in the next few chapters.

# RECONNECTING WITH NATURE

When it comes to treating the whole person, don't underestimate the importance of environment. Bonneteau asks her patients whether they are spending enough time in nature. The need to interact with the natural world outside—to spend time in the sunshine with trees and other plants—is often overlooked in our busy and overly frenetic modern lives. It seems that everything we do is increasingly focused on spending time inside, and this simply isn't good for us, explains Bonneteau.

"We've become an indoor species now, living in our houses," Bonneteau says. "We don't go outside; instead we're playing video games, watching movies, sitting on the sofa. We're not designed for that. Basically, we're designed to be outdoors and in the sunshine." On the whole, humans function optimally when we spend time outdoors getting sunlight, fresh air, and interacting with the natural world. Bonneteau says that nurturing our connection with nature is a critical element in healing eczema and plays a key role in restoring our overall health and wellness.

And certainly, medical science has long noted that spending time outside has significant and wide-ranging health benefits. One study published in 2018 looked at the data of 290 million people and found that populations with higher levels of green-space exposure were more likely to report good overall health.

This may be especially true for people with eczema. As noted in Chapter 3, exposing your skin to sunlight can help diminish an eczema flare. This is the idea behind phototherapy, which has been proven to be an effective treatment for moderate to severe eczema. Spending time outside can also help balance our circadian rhythm, or the daily cycle we naturally follow for when we're active, when we eat, and when we rest. This natural rhythm lets our bodies know when to settled down and sleep. Having a set sleeping pattern can be helpful for people with eczema who struggle to sleep during flares, Bonneteau explains.

"A lot of my work is about reconnecting people with the nature that's around them. And just doing that makes a huge difference," Bonneteau says. She recommends simply taking a half-hour walk. "If you can do that a few times in the week, you'll feel so much better."

## DO ALTERNATIVE TREATMENTS WORK?

This is the million-dollar question. There's no clear answer because treatments are individualized, so what works for one person may not work for another.

Holistic providers such as Cameron and Bonneteau believe that alternative treatments can be highly effective. Bonneteau says that her practices have helped her heal from the inside out. Slowly but surely, she says, her eczema is leaving her body. She doesn't use creams anymore, and her horrible hay fever and seasonal allergies are gone, she says. At times she has a bit of redness on the tops of her fingers, but at other times she'll go up to six months without any eczema at all.

The problem, critics say, is that rigorous clinical trials for complementary and alternative medicine are often lacking. Research and studies into the effectiveness of an alternative treatment are often small and poorly controlled. Some researchers note that when they have attempted to do a review of literature on alternative practices, they have found that there is simply insufficient evidence of the practice or treatment's effectiveness.

Alternative treatments aren't really conducive to that kind of large-scale investigation. Many of these treatments are not standardized; each practitioner may have a slightly different way of approaching a treatment. The same goes for herbal remedies and natural or alternative products. The formulations of products, or protocols for how to use them, can vary widely. This makes it hard to do large-scale, evidence-based studies. Instead the evaluation of a therapy often comes down to anecdotal information and word of mouth from others who have tried it.

Overall, the effects of many alternative treatments are modest, but most treatments have few side effects and are relatively affordable, Lio notes. More people are using alternative approaches, and they will likely continue to do so, especially when conventional approaches aren't getting the job done. Picking the right alternative treatment is going to take trying out different things out to see what fits for you.

# CHAPTER 7

# ECZEMA AND NUTRITION

Food is often one of the first culprits that people blame when it comes to eczema. Many people believe that diet is a root cause of their eczema, which spurs them to examine their dietary habits, and sometimes make sweeping changes in hopes of finding the key to getting their skin under control. Given the close association between eczema and food allergies, it's no wonder that people often feel that their diet can have real impacts on their skin, either contributing to eczema flare-ups or helping to calm things down.

But the exact influence of food on eczema remains unclear, and the scientific data on what type of diet is best for limiting flare-ups and helping to clear eczema is at best mixed. It's been shown that people tend to blame food and diet for their flare-ups but that once their eczema symptoms are under control, those associations are often dropped. One interesting study, conducted by Michele Thompson and Jon Hanifin, found that in 80 percent of cases in which patients were convinced that food was a significant factor contributing to their eczema, such concerns became negligible once better control of the eczema was achieved.

Of course, a simple internet search will return mounds of online articles and blogs that give firsthand accounts of how dietary changes (either incorporating or excluding certain foods) seemed to help "cure" a person's eczema. But what's not clear is how successful everyone else will be if they follow that same diet. And most importantly, will that diet work for you?

Many nutritionists and holistic practitioners believe that proper nutrition and diet is key to support healing from the inside out. We know that what we eat plays a crucial role in many aspects of our health, including that of our skin. But what, exactly, is the best diet to follow has long been a topic of debate, and the picture is just as murky when it comes to figuring out which diet is best for eczema. Dietary recommendations can run the gamut and will vary greatly depending on a practitioner's approach.

Like most things when it comes to eczema, while one thing seems to work well for one person, the complete opposite may work well for another. Below we'll look at some of the main theories swirling around diet and eczema, along with several ways that nutritionists and practitioners approach food as part of their healing practices for eczema.

## THE LEAKY GUT

Is it possible that a chronic disease like eczema may actually be rooted in problems with the intestines? That eczema is really "leaky skin," and what is happening on the outside is probably mirrored on the inside? This is the theory behind the "leaky gut," or intestinal hyperpermeability, a condition that many nutritionists and holistic and alternative practitioners associate with eczema and atopic diseases.

As naturopath and nutritionist Rebecca Bonneteau explains, leaky gut syndrome takes into account the idea that people with eczema have a skin barrier dysfunction that impairs the skin's ability to retain moisture. This dysfunction means the skin becomes overly dry, which contributes to the development of eczema. As was mentioned in previous chapters, immunologists also believe that dry, inflamed eczematous skin is a risk factor in young children developing food allergies and other allergic diseases. Researchers believe that children who are exposed to certain food proteins (specifically peanut proteins) through broken skin can become sensitized to these foods and develop food allergies.

As Bonneteau explains it, people with eczema have leaky, broken skin that is letting particles through and causing the immune system to react in a skewed way. It's not hard to imagine that if your skin is broken and inflamed on the outside, you may also be dealing with similar issues on the inside. The gastrointestinal tract is essentially a long tube made up of tissues that secrete digestive hormones and extract and absorb nutrients and water as food is digested. The theory of leaky gut syndrome is that if the lining of the intestines is inflamed and damaged, it can cause a barrier dysfunction, allowing food particles, bacteria, and toxins to escape into the bloodstream. A leaky gut may be contributing to skewed immune responses, worsening your eczema or causing you to become sensitized to certain foods, Bonneteau explains. This is one of the reasons why holistic and alternative healers often focus on food, nutrition, and healing your gut if you have eczema.

However, conventional medicine considers leaky gut syndrome to be a hypothetical condition that hasn't been definitively proven to exist. Many physicians believe that this condition is more myth than reality. Still, some physicians are intrigued by the leaky gut hypothesis, especially in light of what we know about eczema and skin barrier dysfunction, says Dr. Peter Lio.

There is some evidence to suggest that what is happening in our intestines may be correlated to what is happening on our skin, notes Lio. We know that food can be a trigger for some people with eczema and that food allergies are closely linked to eczema. We also know that there is a great deal of interaction between our immune systems and the bacteria in our gut. And there is much research going on in the medical world to examine and better understand the interplay between the microbiome in our gut and its impact on many aspects of our health. More research is needed to fully study and understand this theory, but many holistic practitioners, including Bonneteau, say they believe they already have the answers.

## TRACKING FOOD, MOOD, AND POOP

The first step to understanding how food may be impacting your eczema and overall health is to get a better picture of how you are interacting with food. From a holistic perspective, diet and nutrition are key factors in healing yourself from the inside out. The first step to doing this is to pay attention to not only the role that food is playing in your overall health, but also your feelings and emotions surrounding your diet and how you eat, notes Cameron. This is why Cameron and other practitioners often advise patients to begin tracking their food, bodily functions, and reactions (both physical and emotional) to what they eat. This is what Cameron calls a "food, mood, and poop journal." Cameron shared her experience as a holistic practitioner treating people with eczema, as well as her own experience in dealing with eczema, during her phone interview.

Tracking all of these things can also help you see the bigger picture of how food affects you and the power it has over you, explains Cameron. Many people have a complicated relationship with food, and what we eat can be tied to how we feel. Understanding how we interact with food can also help you pick a diet that you'll be able to stick with. It's easy to say that you'll make changes to your diet, such as only eating certain healthy foods, but being on a strict diet can make you feel deprived, which can lead you to rebound and eat foods that aren't good for you.

"I want people to notice their patterning around foods, notice what your relationship is to food, and how you're feeling around food," Cameron says. "Notice when you binge or when you eat to kill time, and notice if there's any triggering around that."

## ARE FOOD ALLERGENS TRIGGERING FLARE-UPS?

Because food allergies are considered to be closely associated with eczema, food allergens are often one of the first things people look into when it comes to diet and eczema. However, it's important to remember that there is a difference between having a food allergy and having a food sensitivity or intolerance, says Lio. A food allergy provokes an immune response (which in some cases can be dangerous or life-threatening). A food sensitivity or intolerance may leave you with uncomfortable symptoms such as bloating, gastric pain, and diarrhea. For some people with inflammatory diseases like eczema, a food intolerance or sensitivity may cause an "eczematous" reaction. But these reactions can take hours or even days to appear, so it can also be really hard to identify which foods are causing this reaction. Also, many people notice that these reactions seem to diminish once they get their eczema under control, notes Lio.

Still, many people begin to explore the link between their diet and their eczema by looking at common food allergens. These often include the top eight food allergens, which are the most common foods that people are allergic to:

- Gluten and wheat
- Milk and dairy products
- Eggs
- Peanuts
- Soy and soy products
- Fish
- Shellfish
- Tree nuts (such as almonds, walnuts, and pistachios)

The next step many people take is to try an elimination diet to see exactly what foods seem to be triggering their eczema. People often begin an elimination diet with the common food allergens.

## FINDING YOUR FOOD TRIGGERS WITH AN ELIMINATION DIET

An elimination diet is one way to determine whether you have food sensitivities or food intolerances that may be triggering your eczema. You should never conduct an elimination diet to determine a food allergy on your own—any reintroduction of such a food you know you're allergic to should be done under the supervision of a medical professional.

Currently, there is dispute about the specific mechanisms that cause us to react to foods, and it can be difficult to identify these suspected food culprits. However, according to the University of Wisconsin–Madison School of Medicine and Public Health's UW Integrative Health Program, an elimination diet is one of the best tools for identifying food culprits and is very safe, as long as a variety of foods are still eaten so that you are still getting essential nutrients while eliminating other foods.

Before you begin an elimination diet, it's always a good idea to consult your health-care provider. Also, consider whether this is a good time to undertake such a major change in your diet. If you're in the middle of stressful life event or challenges, or just getting ready for holiday celebrations or a big vacation, you may want to wait until your daily life seems more stable before taking on an elimination diet.

Most elimination diets begin by having you make a list of all the foods you suspect may be a problem. Consider what foods you eat most often and what foods you crave. Pay attention to the timing of any reactions you may have. If you have a food allergy, you'll likely have a reaction right away, but a reaction caused by a food sensitivity or intolerance can take several hours, or even up to two days. Besides eczema flares, other symptoms to be on the lookout for include stomach and bowel irritation, headaches, hives, itching, and generally feeling unwell.

Identifying foods you may be sensitive to can be tricky. Sometimes it's a specific compound in the food that causes the reaction, so you always have a negative reaction every time you eat it, but sometimes a sensitivity is triggered only when you eat too much of one type of food, or if you eat different foods with the same compound. It may be that your body can tolerate a certain amount of a food, but once you reach a threshold or a tipping point, your symptoms return.

This is why it's important to remove all the possible foods that may be causing you a problem. You'll need to stop eating those foods for several weeks (UW Integrative Health recommends starting with two weeks). You'll also need to check all food labels and be careful when eating out to make sure you don't inadvertently end up eating one of the foods you are eliminating.

If your symptoms haven't improved in two weeks, UW Integrative Health recommends continuing for up to four weeks. If your symptoms haven't improved in four weeks, stop the diet. You can then try again with a different set of foods. If an elimination diet doesn't work for you, you may wish to try a different diet.

## TESTING YOUR BODY WITH FOOD CHALLENGES

If your symptoms improve with the elimination diet, wait until you're symptom-free for at least five days before beginning the next phase: food challenges. This entails systematically challenging your body by slowly reintroducing the foods you removed back into your diet one at a time. As you do this, track any symptoms. By reintroducing foods slowly and methodically you'll be able to get a clearer picture of what, exactly, you're reacting to. You'll want to add a new food back into your diet every three days or so. Some elimination diets suggest that after reintroducing a food, you go back to the full elimination diet for a couple of days so you can better assess how you feel.

A word of caution: food challenges for foods you are sensitive or intolerant to can cause severe reactions in people who are highly sensitive to different foods. If you're at risk for such a reaction, you may wish to discuss an elimination diet with your healthcare provider beforehand. You should not attempt to reintroduce foods you already know you are allergic to, as food allergies can cause anaphylaxis. Once again, food challenges for a true food allergy should only be done under the close supervision of an experienced practitioner in a setting that's properly equipped to deal with potentially severe allergic reactions.

Once you have identified the foods you have an intolerance or sensitivity to, you can remove those from your diet altogether, or you may be able to eat those foods on occasion, depending on how well or how often your body can tolerate them. Some people may find they are able to tolerate eating small amounts of foods they are sensitive to.

## ELIMINATION DIETS DON'T WORK FOR EVERYONE

Keep in mind that elimination diets do come with some potential downfalls. Lio has seen many patients who have tried elimination diets only to end up even more frustrated and without any new information or answers as to what is causing their eczema. For one thing, it may be hard to determine the cause of an eczema flare after a food challenge because of how long it may take for some of these reactions to happen. We still don't have a very good understanding of how or why people react to certain foods.

Elimination diets often severely restrict what you can eat for a period of time, and for a lot of people they don't work, Lio says. Another concern is that elimination diets may not provide you with a good balance of nutrition. In some patients, especially children, this could lead to malnutrition, Lio notes. This is why elimination diets are never meant to be sustained for a long period of time.

From a naturopathic perspective, Bonneteau says she is also wary of strict elimination diets. Even if a person does feel some relief from the diet, an elimination diet isn't going to fix the root problem of what is causing the eczema. And because you can't stay on an elimination diet forever, those who do find relief from removing those foods may find they feel even worse when they try to reintroduce those foods again, Bonneteau explains. Once a food you are sensitive to is reintroduced, it can be a shock to the system for some, and the symptoms can feel heightened.

Instead of eliminations diets, Lio recommends focusing on repairing the skin barrier, because "leaky skin" can contribute to the development of allergies, especially in young children. He likens using an elimination diet to the idea that "if your house keeps getting broken into, one solution is to try to get rid of all the bad guys in the world. Another is to simply secure your house against bad guys, which is a lot more tenable."

## DIET MAY OFFER ANSWERS WHEN NOTHING ELSE HELPS

However, elimination diets have been widely used by both conventional and holistic practitioners for a number of reasons, and some people report that they have been helpful. For example, Jennifer Roberge, whose son had severe eczema as a young child, says that modern medicine seemed to have few tools to help her manage her son's eczema. Roberge is the founder of The Eczema Company, which features natural skin care and alternative products. She isn't a holistic practitioner herself, but she has worked with different holistic practitioners and has researched a number of alternative treatments for eczema. Conventional physicians didn't have any other therapies to offer beyond prescribing stronger and stronger topical corticosteroids. She also felt that there was a strong connection between her son's flares and the type of food he was eating.

Frustrated and fed up with conventional medicine, Roberge eventually had her son do several different elimination diets. Watching his skin clear and then seeing distinct reactions to different foods as they were reintroduced was helpful in determining what food sensitivities were triggering eczema in her son. The elimination diet helped her determine that a gluten sensitivity, in combination with other foods, seemed to be causing the bulk of his flares.

Roberge says she uses a four-day rotation diet with her son now that she knows his food triggers. With this diet, he can eat foods he is sensitive to every four days, which allows him to have exposure to all different foods. However, his body is able to handle these foods when they are spaced out, and this greatly diminishes how often food triggers his eczema.

## REDUCING FOOD TRIGGERS WITH A LOW-HISTAMINE DIET

Another option some people find helpful in reducing food triggers is to reduce or eliminate foods that have high histamine levels. The idea is that you may have a histamine intolerance, so eating foods high in histamine may trigger an allergy-like response. There isn't a lot of data to show how widespread this might be, but one small study looked at the impact of a low-histamine diet on 36 people with eczema. The study found that 30 percent of those patients benefited from a histamine-free diet with improved eczema. High-histamine foods include the following:

- Alcohol
- Fermented foods such as sauerkraut
- Hard cured sausages
- Smoked meat products such as salami, ham, and sausage

- Shellfish
- Beans and legumes, such as soybeans, peanuts, and chickpeas
- Nuts, such as walnuts and cashews
- Chocolate and cocoa-based products

There are also "histamine-liberating foods," which are known to help release histamines in other foods. Histamine-liberating foods include the following:

- Most citrus fruits, including lemon and lime (although some may be well tolerated)
- Pineapple, kiwi, and strawberries
- Tomatoes
- Nuts
- Chocolate
- Beans and legumes

In addition, certain foods are believed to help reduce inflammation. Some foods contain quercetin, a powerful antioxidant and antihistamine that can help reduce inflammation. Quercetin is also an ingredient found in a number of herbal remedies and supplements. Foods high in quercetin include the following:

- Apples
- Blueberries
- Cherries
- Broccoli
- Spinach
- Kale
- Onions

# WHOLE FOODS FOR WHOLE SKIN

Many experts believe that eating foods as close to their natural form as possible is generally a healthier option. This is called a "whole foods diet" or "eating clean," and it focuses on fresh, unprocessed, nutritious foods. A whole foods diet promotes eating foods such as fruits, vegetables, beans, chicken, and seafood. It advocates choosing whole grains over refined grains and avoiding processed foods with additives such as sugar, fat, flavorings, or preservatives.

The whole foods diet looks to reduce the consumption of prepared, ready-to-eat foods—basically nixing foods that come in a package or that are sold in a vending machine. The idea is that artificial flavorings, sugars, and chemical additives introduce toxins to the body that are generally unhealthy. And for someone dealing with chronic eczema, they may be triggering flares.

## PLANT-BASED FOODS TO FIGHT ECZEMA

Some believe a plant-based diet of fruits and vegetables helps to reduce eczema flares. Many people also opt to skip dairy because of its potential inflammatory effects. One small study conducted in Sweden monitored 24 people with severe asthma who were put on a strict plant-based vegan diet. At the end of four months, 71 percent saw improvement in their symptoms.

Bonneteau says that if patients are willing to try it, adopting a plant-based diet can be very healing for the skin and the gut. She also recommends skipping dairy and meat, which she believes are often inflammatory or mucus-creating. Bonneteau emphasizes eating "soothing foods" such as smoothies and juices, which are packed with nutrient-dense fruits and vegetables. She likens smoothies and juices to using moisturizers and cream on your skin to soothe and calm it down. A smoothie can work the same way, hydrating the body from the inside, Bonneteau explains.

# CARNIVORE-BASED DIET TO SPEED HEALING

It is an extreme approach, but some claim to have found success with an all-meat diet. This diet has been gaining some traction as a possible anti-inflammatory diet for people with autoimmune conditions. It's promoted by Mikhaila Peterson, a Canadian social media star who shares dietary plans on her blog, *Don't Eat That*. Some holistic nutritionists consider this an extreme elimination diet to remove any food sensitives.

Although it might sound strange to some, eating an all-meat diet has been helping in reducing itching and other eczema symptoms, says East Asian medicine practitioner Tara Cameron. Cameron, who has also experienced topical steroid withdrawal, says she was a little surprised when she switched to an all-meat diet and found it helped her skin heal, among other benefits. She acknowledges that this strict diet may not be for everyone and that it can be hard to maintain. To make sure she gets the nutrition she needs, she includes a variety of organ meat and fish in her diet.

It's important to note that there is no research or clinical data on the effectiveness of an all-meat diet. It also raises various concerns, one of which is that such a restrictive, unbalanced diet may not meet a person's dietary needs.

# GLUTEN-FREE DIETS

In recent years, gluten- and wheat-free diets have come into the spotlight, even for people who are not gluten-sensitive. Many nutritionists and holistic medicine practitioners believe that wheat and gluten may trigger eczema. Bonneteau says she often recommends removing wheat and gluten because these foods are considered irritating, especially if a person is suspected to have a leaky gut.

A few conditions are known to be triggered by wheat and gluten. One rare disease, dermatitis herpetiformis, is associated with celiac disease and is an example of a gluten-associated skin disorder, explains Lio. Some patients may have symptoms that look like eczema, including itchy bumps and small blisters on reddish skin. Sometimes these patients may even be misdiagnosed with eczema.

There may also be an association between celiac disease and eczema, although a causal relationship has not been established. A 2004 study that looked at 1,000 patients with celiac disease found they were three times as likely to have eczema than the general population. However, even after being on a gluten-free diet for a year, their eczema symptoms hadn't improved.

A literature review of controlled trials had similar findings. It found that gluten was among those foods that may cause nonallergy-driven inflammation in some patients, which may lead to the worsening of eczema in some people. But the study went on to say that these associations weren't clearly defined and that most people who avoided gluten for one year didn't see improvements in eczema flares.

Overall, there isn't a lot of data to support avoiding gluten, but some people may find from personal experience that gluten can trigger their eczema.

## EATING A WELL-BALANCED DIET

Some people with eczema have found that certain diets make them feel better and seem to reduce their symptoms. Finding the right diet means paying close attention to the foods you eat and seeing if you have any symptoms. But in general, most dietitians recommend eating a well-balanced diet. One example of this is the Mediterranean diet, which emphasizes fruits, vegetables, cereals, fish, and healthy fats such as olive oil. Many of these foods are known to have anti-inflammatory properties.

Although there is not a lot of data looking at the Mediterranean diet and eczema, one 2018 study found that it may improve psoriasis, another inflammatory skin disease that can be triggered by environmental factors. Researchers found that those who ate a Mediterranean diet were less likely to have severe cases of the disease.

# CHAPTER 8

# EVERYDAY NATURAL APPROACHES TO TREATING ECZEMA

Humans have been using natural remedies for thousands of years, and even in this age of modern medicine, this trend shows no sign of stopping. Taking a simple, natural approach to supporting and healing your skin makes a lot of sense. Plus, most of these topicals and supplements are easily found at local stores or online, and many may be more affordable than prescription medications, which seem to be rising in cost every year.

Many natural remedies have been shown to be effective, and some of them can be quite powerful. But before you begin swallowing supplements or slathering on natural botanical moisturizers, let's take a closer look at these options—what has been shown to work, and what hasn't? While natural products can have a range of benefits, one potential drawback is that there is often a lack of data and clinical studies to show how effective such approaches are.

Modern medicine has more answers than ever before, but there are still significant gaps in our knowledge when it comes to natural remedies for eczema, says Dr. Peter Lio, founding director of the Chicago Integrative Eczema Center. So it's important to let your health-care provider know about any supplements and natural remedies you're using, as some may have interactions with other medications you are taking.

## CARING FOR YOUR SKIN THE NATURAL WAY

Pretty packaging and fancy brands don't necessarily add up to more effective skin care. Sometimes natural products can include surprising and hidden benefits, without the concerns of using harmful chemicals. However, you should do a patch test before using a new product, especially if you're prone to reactions or have sensitive skin.

One simple way to do a patch test is to apply a small amount of product to the inside of your wrist or to the side of your neck, because these areas have thinner, more delicate skin. Cover the area with a bandage and wait 24 hours to see if you have a reaction. If you have any questions, consult your health-care provider.

This chapter looks in depth at a number of natural topicals that are believed to help with eczema and examines some of the research behind their effectiveness.

**Coconut Oil**—This natural emollient has long been considered a safe way to soften and soothe the skin. Coconut oil can help reduce irritation and itching, and researchers have found that it has a number of other health benefits, Lio notes. Coconut oil is rich in lauric acid, a fatty acid that randomized controlled trials have found can decrease staph colonization by 95 percent in patients with eczema. A 2018 study found that coconut oil has anti-inflammatory properties, and a 2014 scientific review found that it can effectively reduce the presence of bacteria, viruses, and fungi.

However, some people with eczema report that coconut oil isn't moisturizing enough for their skin, or that they are prone to react to it, so be sure to patch test it first.

**Sunflower Seed Oil**—This oil is rich in linoleic acid, a fatty acid that is believed to play a role in maintaining the skin barrier and decreasing the amount of water we lose from our skin. Maintaining the skin's natural moisture is crucial to managing eczema.

The evidence shows that sunflower seed oil has at least a modest effect on chronic eczema, notes Lio. One study showed that children with moderate eczema who used a cream containing sunflower seed oil, along with a topical corticosteroid, had decreased leathery patches of skin and less skin damage from itching and scratching. They also ended up using less corticosteroids and reported an improved quality of life.

**Topical Vitamin B12**—Also known as cobalamin, this topical vitamin is considered to be a compelling addition to the natural arsenal against eczema, Lio explains. Some studies have found that applying vitamin B12 to the skin decreases eczema symptoms by reducing the production of nitric oxide, which has been linked to triggering itch in people with chronic eczema.

At least two randomized controlled trials have found that applying cream containing vitamin B12 has been effective in helping to reduce multiple symptoms of eczema.

**Honey**—Natural healers have long recognized honey's healing powers; for centuries they have been using the sticky bee-made substance as a natural antibacterial and anti-inflammatory agent to heal wounds. It's believed that manuka honey in particular possesses wound-healing properties. Manuka honey is made by bees that collect the pollen from the manuka tree, also known as the tea tree. Tea tree has also been used for centuries for its wound-healing abilities.

Manuka honey contains a number of natural chemicals that are believed to aid its ability to shorten healing time. When used for medical purposes, honey needs to be sterilized by gamma irradiation, which does not have any impact on antibacterial activity. One review of medical literature published in *Jundishapur Journal of Natural Pharmaceutical Products* in August 2013 noted that "honey has almost equal or slightly superior effects when compared with conventional treatments for acute wounds and superficial partial thickness burns."

Another small study found that patients who used manuka honey on eczema lesions nightly for a week saw more healing and had significantly lower severity of symptoms on the lesions where the honey was used, versus other areas that were not treated with honey.

Jennifer Roberge says she has used manuka honey with good success and recommends to others. "We love organic manuka cream. I use it on all of my kids," Roberge says. "We find that it's wound healing. The product we use is between a balm and a cream, and it doesn't burn or sting."

**Tea Tree Oil**—Chances are you've at least heard of tea tree oil, an essential oil made from the leaves of the tea tree (Melaleuca alternifolia). This oil is used in many skin-care products and can be used for medicinal purposes, including treating a variety of skin disorders. A 2013 review found that the oil has anti-inflammatory, antibacterial, and wound-healing properties.

Some of the potential benefits for eczema include reducing inflammation, helping to heal infected skin, and even reducing skin hypersensitivity to some skin allergens and irritants such as nickel. Tea tree oil has antifungal properties and can help reduce specific yeasts that are known to cause dandruff or seborrheic dermatitis; it can also help reduce itching on the scalp.

However, before you use tea tree oil, make sure it is diluted in a carrier oil and do a patch test to make sure your skin doesn't negatively react to it. Some people may be allergic or sensitive to this oil.

## DAILY SUPPLEMENTS FOR HEALTHIER SKIN

Many of us take over-the-counter supplements in the hopes that these vitamins, minerals, or herbal products will help improve our health. And supplements can be helpful in filling in gaps in our diet and providing nutrients we may be deficient in. But supplements can also have powerful unintended effects on the body and can trigger other health problems if they aren't used correctly. Or they may do nothing and have little to no effect in preventing your eczema flare-ups.

So what does the evidence and research show when it comes to how supplements may enhance your well-being when you're battling eczema? Let's take a closer look at some supplements that may be helpful and some that you may want to skip.

**Probiotics**—These are microorganisms, or live bacteria and yeast, that are the same or similar to those found naturally throughout your body, including on your skin and in your digestive system. Researchers have theorized that the way our gut microbiome is colonized when we are babies influences the development of our immune system. This theory has prompted several studies to look at the potential uses of oral probiotics. One such study found that probiotics helped reduce the development of chronic eczema in babies and children, with half as many children developing chronic eczema than the placebo group.

However, other studies have had conflicting results, and major questions still remain, Lio explains. It's still unclear what strain of probiotics is best to use, and at what dosage and frequency probiotics are most effective. Lio says that in his experience with patients, probiotics haven't seemed to help, but they also haven't seemed to hurt. Ultimately, he says, he leaves it to his patients to decide for themselves.

In addition to oral probiotics, some researchers are also looking into whether applying topical probiotics can improve the skin's barrier function and whether that can help reduce the severity of eczema symptoms. Some initial studies look promising, but more research is needed.

**Vitamin D**—We know that eczema tends to be more prevalent in regions located at higher latitudes. One theory is that there may be a link between having lower levels of vitamin D and an increased risk of developing eczema. Medical literature reviews have found that people living in northern latitudes are at higher risk for vitamin D deficiencies, especially during the winter when there is limited sunlight in these areas. This is one of the reasons why vitamin D supplements may be helpful to some people. Cameron, who lives and practices in the Seattle, Washington, area (in the Pacific Northwest region of the US), says she often recommends this supplement to her patients with eczema.

There is limited but compelling data on vitamin D's effectiveness as a supplement that could benefit people with eczema, explains

Lio. A small but impressive study found that vitamin D could be helpful in decreasing the severity of chronic eczema, especially during winter months, when we may not be getting as much vitamin D naturally through sunlight exposure, Lio notes.

Zinc—This mineral is crucial for many metabolic reactions in the body. The skin contains the body's third-largest store of zinc, and the mineral is believed to play an important role in skin barrier function. However, we still don't understand the exact relationship between zinc and eczema.

A review of 16 studies found that low zinc levels in hair and red blood cells were associated with eczema, but better-quality studies are needed to confirm this as well as to evaluate the effectiveness of zinc supplements in treating or preventing eczema.

Another option is to simply boost the amount of zinc you get from your diet. Zinc-rich foods include oysters, grass-fed beef, lamb, sesame and pumpkin seeds, chickpeas, lentils, cashews, spinach, asparagus, and mushrooms.

Collagen—Some people heap a spoonful of collagen powder into their morning coffee or other beverage in hopes of smoothing out wrinkles and keeping joints limber. Collagen is sometimes called the body's scaffolding because it acts like the glue that holds the body together. Collagen makes up 80 percent of the skin and works with elastin to keep the skin supple and stretchable. Cameron recommends collagen supplements for patients with eczema because it's believed to help skin heal and repair itself.

However, the few studies that have been done on the effectiveness of collagen supplements have been small and funded by companies that make these products, increasing the chance of bias. There seems to be some evidence that collagen supplements may help support skin and increase overall hydration, but better-quality studies are needed.

**Quercetin**—This is an antioxidant contained in various foods, including apples, berries, grapes, broccoli, spinach, kale, and onions, as well as in green tea and red wine. It has been found to have immune-modulating and anti-inflammatory properties, which means that quercetin can act as a natural antihistamine and may be helpful in decreasing itch, Cameron notes. Quercetin has been shown to effectively inhibit the secretion of histamine and pro-inflammatory markers, and it may help decrease eczema that has not responded to conventional treatments.

**Licorice Root Extract**—This herb is commonly used in many Traditional Chinese Medicine remedies. It may be helpful if you are having an acute eczema flare, because it can provoke a cortical response in the body similar to taking corticosteroids, says Cameron. The herb's key therapeutic compound, glycyrrhizin (glycyrrhizinic acid), seems to prevent the breakdown of adrenal hormones such as cortisol (the body's primary stress-fighting adrenal hormone), making these hormones more available to the body. It has also been found that licorice cream, applied directly to irritated skin, can help to reduce inflammation and relieve symptoms such as itching and burning and can also boost the effectiveness of cortisone creams. One double-blind clinical trial found that glycyrrhizinic acid in a 2 percent topical formulation helped control itching and could be considered an effective treatment for chronic eczema.

Licorice root may be effective against bacteria that can infect the skin, according to a study in the *Iranian Journal of Pharmaceutical Research*. That study showed antimicrobial activity against

Staphylococcus aureus, which can cause skin infections such as impetigo, cellulitis, and folliculitis, which people with eczema may be more prone to develop.

However, licorice root is also known to have some side effects and should be used with caution. Cameron notes that licorice should be avoided if you have high blood pressure. Some studies have also found that pregnant women should avoid licorice. For instance, a 2009 study found that glycyrrhizin in licorice could harm the developing brain of a fetus, and an older study found that heavy licorice consumption could lead to preterm birth.

Because licorice can have a similar action in the body as corticosteroids, Cameron also doesn't recommend this supplement if you are going through topical steroid withdrawal, since the process requires you to wean off of corticosteroids.

**Evening Primrose Oil and Borage Oil**—According to Lio, both evening primrose and borage oils have been believed to benefit the skin barrier and to possess anti-inflammatory and anti-itch properties. But when put to the test, the data for both was inconclusive. In fact, one report concluded that taking borage oil and evening primrose orally had the same effect as placebos in trials.

Evening primrose oil, when taken orally, is thought to have a stabilizing effect on the skin barrier, which could make it effective in treating signs and symptoms of eczema. Evening primrose oil is rich in gamma-linolenic acid, a fatty acid that's normally found in healthy skin. Researchers hypothesize that people with eczema often have a skin barrier dysfunction, and it's believed that this dysfunction impedes the skin's ability to convert certain enzymes into the gamma-linoleic acid it needs to function property. So, hypothetically, an oral dose of evening primrose oil may be just the thing the skin needs to stay healthy.

One small study of 65 children and adults found that taking 2,000 to 6,000 milligrams of evening primrose oil orally helped reduce itching and the intensity of symptoms when compared with a placebo.

Derived from the seeds of the flowering herb borage (Borago officinalis), borage oil is rich with omega-6 essential fatty acids and has two to three times more gamma-linolenic acid than evening primrose oil. A review of 12 clinical trials that used borage oil to treat or prevent eczema showed mixed results. Five of the studies reviewed indicated significant improvements for patients who used borage oil, while five others showed insignificant improvement, and two other studies were inconclusive.

## TURN YOUR BATH INTO A HEALING OASIS

Bathing and prolonged soaking in the tub is often encouraged by dermatologists as a way to increase the amount of water and moisture in the skin and to help strengthen the skin barrier. Not surprisingly, many people with eczema enjoy using different additives in their bathwater that may offer therapeutic benefits.

Of course, if you're dealing with eczema, you should be careful to avoid products that are possible irritants, such as fragrances, colorants, or other ingredients that might be irritating to your skin. The bathing therapies that are believed to do the most good usually seem to have an antibacterial or anti-inflammatory effect on the skin, as this is believed to help fight bacterial skin infections or decrease symptoms such as itchiness and redness.

Here are a few different bathing therapies that you may find helpful.

**Salt Baths**—Many people with eczema say they find relief from itchy skin by adding salts to their baths. In particular, Dead Sea salt is heralded by some for its healing power because it also contains various minerals, including high levels of magnesium, calcium, and bromide. Magnesium is known to help lessen inflammatory diseases and to possess wound-healing properties.

Also, some people report that Epsom salt baths have been a tremendous help in decreasing their eczema, although there's no real data to support this. Like Dead Sea salt, Epsom salt contains magnesium.

**Apple Cider Vinegar**—This is a popular home remedy for many skin disorders. Any type of vinegar may act as an antibacterial and an antifungal. However, apple cider vinegar also contains by-products from fermentation that are believed to promote skin health, help soothe skin infections and irritations, and rebalance the skin's acidity level.

Just keep in mind that apple cider vinegar is highly acidic and should only be used in small amounts as it can burn your skin if not properly diluted. Researchers and doctors have documented cases where people have injured their skin when attempting to use apple cider vinegar. The National Eczema Association recommends adding two cups of apple cider vinegar to a full tub of warm water and then soaking for 15 to 20 minutes, followed by the use of a gentle moisturizer.

Some people also use highly diluted apple cider vinegar in wet body wraps. To use it this way, mix one tablespoon of apple cider vinegar with one cup of warm water. Dip clean cotton fabric, gauze, or paper towels in the mixture and wrap this around the area affected by eczema. Cover with a clean, dry dressing, such as cotton fabric. Wear this wrap for at least three hours or overnight.

**Colloidal Oatmeal**—This is made from oats that have been ground and boiled to extract their skin-healing properties. Soaking in colloidal oatmeal has been found to have soothing properties, probably because it's rich in beta-glucans, which can help reduce skin inflammation and stimulate collagen production. Colloidal oatmeal also helps create a protective barrier against irritants while providing additional nutrients to the skin.

Colloidal oatmeal is generally safe for all ages, but people who are allergic to oats should avoid it. Individuals who are allergic to gluten should also use caution, as oats are often processed on the same equipment as wheat. Studies have found that people who soaked in an oatmeal bath daily saw significant improvements in their eczema. To use, simply add two to three cups of colloidal oatmeal powder to a tub of warm water and soak for up to 15 minutes.

## KEEPING ECZEMA UNDER WRAPS

Eczema can make your skin dry, cracked, and scaly, which is not only painful but also leaves you more exposed to developing a secondary infection. When your skin is in an agonizing flare, it's wise to take extra measures to protect and help your skin heal by covering it up. There are various ways to use wraps and covers to give your skin some extra protection and help it stay moisturized and heal faster.

**Wet Wrapping**—There are many different methods of wet-wrap therapy, with variations in what products and moisturizers are applied to the skin, what type of bandages or dressings are used over the top, how long these are left on, and how frequently the bandages are changed out. Many dermatologists recommend wet-wrapping because it has been found to be an effective short-term treatment and is generally considered safe. Discomfort, such as chills, is the most common adverse side effect of the therapy, notes Lio.

The basic technique of wet wrapping involves first applying a layer of topical medication and/or a moisturizer to dampen skin. Although topical corticosteroids aren't a natural substance, they're often used in wet wrapping, and hydrated skin is able to absorb topical medications better, providing faster relief. Studies have found that using a topical corticosteroid along with a moisturizer is the most effective method, but wet wrapping can also be done with heavy moisturizers alone.

Next, wrap a layer of damp gauze or cloth around the skin, followed by a dry layer of gauze or cloth. Leave all this in place for at least several hours, or overnight. By doing this, Lio explains, you are creating a physical barrier that will help prevent water loss from the skin's surface.

**Dry Wrapping**—While wet wrapping is effective, it can be difficult, especially for young children, who may not like being wrapped up under layers of gauze. Roberge says she used wet wrapping with her son when his eczema was flaring out of control. She found it was an effective way to help give him some relief from severe flares, but she notes that it's not a long-term treatment. Because of some of the drawbacks to wet wrapping, she came up with an alternative wrapping style known as dry wrapping. This is where you apply a layer of moisturizer and wrap with dry cotton clothing. This offers many of the same benefits of wet wrapping, without the discomfort of cold, wet wraps, explains Roberge.

Roberge's experience caring for her son inspired her to launch her own line of breathable garments called Remedywear, which are infused with antibacterial zinc.

# CLOTHING AND FABRICS

The clothes we wear are in contact with our bodies all day long. If you are dealing with chronic eczema, you are probably already aware and careful of what type of clothing and fabric you choose. You likely pay attention to everything from the type of dye used in the cloth to how well the material conducts heat and sweat.

The biggest textile culprit known to contribute to flares is wool. The scratchy, irritating nature of wool means anyone with eczema should steer clear of clothing made with this fiber. But beyond wool avoidance, Lio notes that there is intriguing data about other types of fabrics that may have therapeutic benefits.

**Cotton**—Cotton is the most commonly recommended textile for people with chronic eczema. It is often seen as an eczema-friendly fabric because it's a natural fiber that is soft and breathable. Cotton is generally good at moisture absorption and conducting heat away from the skin.

**Silk**—The super-soft texture of silk feels wonderful against the skin, and the fabric is also known to help maintain body temperature by keeping the wearer cool and reducing excessive sweating and moisture loss, which can worsen dry skin. It's believed that silk may aid in healing rashy skin by enhancing collagen production and decreasing inflammation and the severity of eczemas flares, but conflicting studies cast doubt on that theory.

However, a recent randomized controlled trial that looked at 300 children ages 1 to 15 with moderate to severe eczema found no evidence that wearing silk helped. The study noted that fabrics that have antimicrobial properties may be more helpful.

**Silver-Coated Textiles**—Silver-coated textiles, or silver-impregnated clothing, have been shown to have an antibacterial effect on the skin, especially against Staphylococcus aureus bacteria. Several studies have found that people wearing silver-coated garments showed significant improvement in their eczema over a period of time. One double-blind study found that children with eczema who wore clothing made with seaweed enriched with silver ions improved faster than those who wore standard all-cotton clothes. The author of the study noted that the results also reinforced the importance of non-pharmacological measures, such as clothing, in the management of atopic dermatitis.

## ARE NATURAL PRODUCTS BETTER?

One of the great things about natural products is that most have very few side effects. However, we often have the perception that natural products are inherently better than products that were created in a lab. Natural products may have fewer ingredients, which can be helpful, but you can have reactions to natural ingredients as well as synthetic compounds. Also, some people with eczema and very dry skin complain that natural products aren't as hydrating or don't seem to moisturize the skin as thoroughly as synthetic counterparts. In addition, natural or organic products tend to have a shorter shelf life.

Natural products can have many benefits, one being that you may feel like you can trust a product that has fewer ingredients and potentially health-harming chemicals. They can be used by themselves, or in conjunction with other products or therapies. As with other eczema treatments, you should let your doctor know about any supplements or herbal remedies you are using.

# CHAPTER 9

# BURNING SKIN AND TOPICAL STEROIDS

In 2014 Briana Banos decided to stop using topical steroids to treat her eczema. That one decision changed the course of her life. After years of using topical corticosteroids to manage her eczema flares, she began to realize that something was wrong, and she felt sure it had to do with the amount of topical steroids she had been using. What followed were several years of hell as her skin went through horrific withdrawal symptoms in a condition that is known as topical steroid withdrawal (TSW).

And she's not alone. Banos is among the thousands of people who say they have suffered the effects of TSW. In the last decade, she and others like her have been publicly sharing their TSW stories—often through social media and other online forums. Banos was motivated to do something bigger to raise awareness. She struck on the idea of making a documentary about TSW to delve more deeply into the topic. She raised money through crowdsourcing and spent months traveling the world to interview other patients, their families, and medical experts and physicians who are studying and researching this condition to understand it better.

In March 2019 Banos released her documentary, *Preventable: Protecting Our Largest Organ*, which earned her recognition and acclaim within the eczema community and beyond for her efforts to shed light on this condition. But Banos isn't alone in this fight. A nonprofit group, the International Topical Steroid Addiction Network (ITSAN), says that since it was founded in 2009, it has grown into a worldwide community that provides support and inspiration for TSW sufferers and raises awareness about the condition.

## WHAT IS TSW?

TSW is believed to be a relatively rare side effect of overusing topical steroids. The condition is known by a number of names or descriptors, including red skin syndrome (RSS), topical corticosteroid (TCS) withdrawal, topical steroid addiction (TSA) and topical steroid addiction and withdrawal. Many people who have gone through, or are going through TSW, believe it takes months or years to go through this process, and some feel that TSW may become a chronic condition on its own.

TSW is believed to be caused by the chronic misuse of topical corticosteroids, causing the skin to become addicted or dependent; this is known as topical steroid addiction (TSA). When a person tries to stop using a topical steroid ointment, the skin erupts in a distressing rebound flare that is known as the "rebound effect." This is when the symptoms the topical steroid was intended to treat come back even stronger.

In addition to topical steroids, some patients with eczema may also be prescribed oral steroids. One retrospective cohort study of patients in Australia with symptoms of TSW found that 42 percent of patients had been prescribed an oral corticosteroid for skin symptoms. A history of using oral prednisone for skin issues such as eczema may increase a patient's risk for developing TSW and was considered to be a key factor to be considered when diagnosing TSW, according to a 2018 article published in *Dermatitis*.

Overprescribing topical steroids (such as not requiring mandatory breaks from the drug) or lax monitoring of how often patients refill those prescriptions could be causing more patients to develop TSW, explains Dr. Peter Lio. In a 2019 *Practical Dermatology* journal article, Lio writes that there are two distinct subtypes of TSW:

- **Erythematoedematous**—This tends to affect patients who have chronic eczematous conditions, such as atopic dermatitis. This type is associated with burning, red patches of skin, and swelling.

- **Papulopustular**—This seems to affect people who use topical corticosteroids for cosmetic reasons, such as acne or skin-pigment concerns. Patients with this type have more rosacea-like symptoms, such as papules, pustules, and nodules, and, less frequently, swelling and stinging.

It is believed that TSW can occur within days or weeks of stopping long-term use of topical steroids. Physicians are still trying to understand why this condition develops, but it is generally believed that using stronger or more potent topical steroids for longer periods of time can increase the risk of developing topical steroid addiction. However, it's been noted that even the milder so-called safe topical steroids are not completely without risks when used on a long-term basis. Normal use of topical steroids is not believed to cause TSW, but there can also be differing opinions among physicians as to what, exactly, constitutes "normal use."

Some of the frequently described features of TSW include the following:

- Extremely red, raw-looking skin
- Burning pain and stinging
- Skin sensitivity to previously tolerated skin products
- Excessive peeling and shedding of skin
- Edema, or swelling, especially around the eyes and the ankles
- "Elephant wrinkles," or thickening of the skin with reduced elasticity, such as around elbows or knees
- "Red sleeve," where the arms and/or legs are affected, but the palms and soles of the feet are not
- Headlight sign, in which there is redness of the face but not the nose and around the mouth
- Oozing and weeping skin

In general, using milder topical steroids for a short period of time is considered safe and unlikely to cause problems. However, the definition of "a short period of time" may vary from a few weeks to a few months, depending on the steroid strength and the physician's discretion. But the stronger the topical corticosteroid, and the longer it's used for, the greater the chance of a rebound effect once you stop using it.

It's important to look at bigger trends and patterns in a patient's symptoms and usage, but Lio's rule of thumb is to have patients apply a topical steroid to an area of the body for no more than two weeks per month. That has proven to be a safe approach for most people, and if it isn't working to control symptoms, it's time to look at other options, he says.

Diagnosing TSW can be difficult, because TSW symptoms can be easily mistaken for an eczema flare. Alternatively, an eczema flare can also be mistaken for TSW. Patients who believe their skin is going through withdrawal may avoid using topical steroids, but they may actually be experiencing a flare that needs to be treated, Lio notes.

The concern is that this can lead to a misdiagnosis, which could end up compounding the problem. For instance, patients with a history of long-term use of topical steroids can get caught in a vicious cycle. A patient has an acute flare and is prescribed stronger topical steroids, which create a rebound effect when the treatment ends. The patient may really be having withdrawal symptoms. But it can also appear to worsen the flare symptoms, which could lead to more topical steroids.

This kind of scenario is likely behind many patients' fear and their decision to stop using topical steroids.

## THE DEBATE OVER TSW

In the world of eczema, few topics incite the kind of ire and controversy that topical steroids do. As with most contentious issues, the use and potential overuse of topical steroids is a multifaceted issue, infused with emotion, differing points of view, and a lot of gray areas. But at the heart of the issue are people who feel that the treatment they've been given to manage a chronic condition has actually made their condition much worse, and in some cases has had lasting impacts on their quality of life.

This controversy has created some rifts within the eczema community. Even the medical community has a diversity of opinions and theories about TSW. Some medical experts consider TSW an "emerging" diagnosis, meaning it's a condition that was previously thought to be rare but seems to be rising in prevalence. Some physicians and dermatologists reject the notion of TSW outright or believe that TSW is often simply a severe eczema flare-up—something that should be treated with more potent topical steroids. But TSW advocates argue that such treatments actually worsen this condition.

Many physicians acknowledge that TSW may happen to some patients—after all, it's well documented that chronic overuse of any steroid (topical, inhaled, injected, or oral) can lead to severe side effects. But there may also be other conditions and issues at play behind the TSW condition. On the whole, dermatologists say that TSW itself hasn't been well defined and is not well understood. And most dermatologists stress that topical steroids are a safe and effective treatment in managing eczema.

That doesn't sit well with TSW advocates such as Banos, who say they want to raise the alarm about the potential life-altering harm wrought by the overuse of topical steroids. Some people within the TSW community question whether topical steroids should be used as widely as they are, and whether stricter guidelines are needed to prevent this condition from happening to others. During a phone interview for this book, Banos described her experiences in dealing with eczema and TSW.

"One of the biggest things is that doctors only see what one person is going through, so they negate it, they say it doesn't exist or say it's really rare," says Banos. "That's the reason I wanted to do the documentary, to showcase TSW, so doctors couldn't keep pushing this to the side. I wanted to have proof, to have stories, research, and medical voices all in one film. My main goal is awareness and education but honestly I also hope this kick-starts a shift in how topical steroids are utilized in the medical community."

Meanwhile, the medical and dermatology communities are immersed in their own debate over how to handle TSW. Physicians are trying to understand TSW and how to best work with patients who believe they are going through this condition. Physicians and health-care professionals say they worry that the growing fear about topical steroids may cause patients to unnecessarily forego using this medication, which is considered safe and effective and has been a mainstay in managing eczema for over 50 years.

One thing is clear: TSW is not a simple condition, and there likely aren't simple answers on how to handle it, explains Dr. Jonathan Silverberg, professor of dermatology, director of clinical research, and director of patch testing for the George Washington University School of Medicine's Department of Dermatology. In a phone interview for this book, Silverberg discussed the controversy surrounding topical steroids.

"Topical steroid withdrawal is a very sensitive topic. It evokes a lot of emotions out of a lot of people," says Silverberg. "There's a lot of hype against topical steroids, but the overwhelming majority of patients tolerate them. I don't think there's a universal treatment for everyone, but topical steroids aren't the devil, either."

## TOPICAL STEROIDS: A MIRACLE DRUG?

Our adrenal glands naturally produce a steroid hormone called cortisol, which has a number of functions within our bodies, one of which is to suppress inflammation and alter the immune response. Corticosteroids are synthetic, or manufactured, versions that mimic natural hormones such as cortisol. Topical corticosteroids are used to help reduce skin inflammation by preventing cells from producing inflammation-causing chemicals that are released in response to a variety of different triggers.

When hydrocortisone was discovered in 1952, it was heralded as a kind of miracle drug, ushering in an exciting chapter in dermatological therapy, according to a *Canadian Medical Association Journal* editorial published in January 1973. For the first time, dermatologists had a way to combat rampant skin eruptions and inflammation. "Only those who have faced the frustration of local therapy in the precorticosteroid era can fully realize what a giant step forward hydrocortisone represented," the article declares. But the same article later goes on to say, "Great advances inevitably create new problems. The topical corticosteroids brought many new problems with them, both local and systemic."

There is no doubt that topical steroids have revolutionized the treatment of many types of chronic skin conditions. In the decades since topical steroids were first developed, they have become the cornerstone for treating chronic eczema and many other skin diseases. Topical steroids aren't a cure for eczema, but in effectively controlling inflammation, they are one of the few tools that physicians have to help control flare-ups and relieve symptoms such as itching. Low-potency versions are readily available over the counter. Nevertheless, these topical ointments are drugs, and they can have severe side effects if not used correctly.

Topical steroids come in different strengths, ranging from mild to very potent. Commonly used topical steroids (corticosteroids) include hydrocortisone, triamcinolone, fluocinonide, and clobetasol. Hydrocortisone is one of the lowest-potency steroid creams available. It can be purchased over the counter in strengths up to 1 percent.

Side effects from topical steroids are more common in higher-potency prescription-strength steroid creams and ointments. Even so, a low-potency steroid could cause side effects such as thinning of the skin if used daily for many consecutive weeks. This is especially true if steroid cream is used on thin, sensitive skin such as the eyelids, genital areas, or the folds of the skin. As a general rule, to minimize the risk of side effects, a patient should use the lowest strength that is effective in managing their symptoms. Very potent steroids should only be used on a short-term basis.

## SIDE EFFECTS OF TOPICAL STEROIDS

Topical steroids are known to have a number of side effects. According to the American Academy of Family Physicians, most of these side effects are rare when topical steroids are used properly. Most side effects are associated with prolonged and excessive use and are localized to the areas of the body where the topical steroid was applied. Side effects can include the following:

- **Skin atrophy,** or thinning of the skin—This is the most common side effect. It causes the skin to look lax, transparent, wrinkled, or shiny. This is usually reversed once steroid use is stopped, but it may take months for the skin to return to its normal thickness.

- **Lichenification,** or thickening of the skin—This is usually caused by scratching and rubbing. Lichenification may create leathery patches on the skin.

- **Striae,** or stretch marks—Striae usually only appear on limited areas of the body (on the upper inner thighs, under the arms, in the groin or armpits, and in the creases of the elbows and knees) and aren't usually permanent.

- **Telangiectasia**—Commonly known as spider veins, these are enlarged blood vessels that can appear as threadlike red lines on the skin.

- **Hypopigmentation,** or a discoloring of the skin—This is when topicals cause areas of the skin to become lighter than your overall skin tone.

- **Hypertrichosis**—This is the localized increase of hair thickness and length. This is considered a rare side effect.

- **Increased risk of skin infection**—Topical corticosteroids may suppress the body's immune response, leading to an increased risk of infection, including secondary skin infections.

- **Steroid-induced rosacea and steroid-induced acne**— This condition can also be called steroid dermatitis, and it can be triggered by the use of topical steroids. Affected areas may become flaming red, covered in pus-filled reddish bumps. If topical steroid use continues, or if the condition is left untreated, the skin may become atrophied and permanently damaged.

Topical steroids can also have systemic adverse effects on multiple organs within the body. These side effects are considered very rare, but babies, children, or elderly patients are more susceptible to systemic adverse effects. These can include the following:

- **Adrenal insufficiency**—Chronic use of corticosteroids can hinder the interaction between the hypothalamus, pituitary gland, and adrenal glands. This can lead to adrenal insufficiency, a condition in which the adrenal glands do not produce adequate amounts of steroid hormones, such as cortisol.

- **Iatrogenic Cushing's syndrome**—This is a form of Cushing's syndrome that occurs in people taking glucocorticoid (also called corticosteroid, or steroid) hormones. It is usually related to prolonged and/or high-dose oral steroid use, but it can occur with chronic use of high-potency topical corticosteroids.

- **Glaucoma and loss of vision**—Repeated use of topical steroids around the eyes or on the eyelids has been known to cause glaucoma. This side effect is rare as long as the hydrocortisone product is used as directed.

- **Avascular necrosis of femoral head**—Avascular necrosis is the death of bone tissue due to a lack of blood supply. The femoral head is the highest part of the thigh bone, or femur. This condition could lead to tiny breaks in the bone and the bone's eventual collapse.

- **Growth impairment in infants and children (still under investigation)**—Researchers have long recognized the growth-inhibiting effects of corticosteroids on children, especially those treated for chronic conditions such as inflammatory bowel disease or asthma.

  Chronic eczema has also been associated with poor growth in some severely affected children, especially those who also have asthma and were using more potent topical steroids. Some studies have noted that babies and young children are at risk of absorbing topically applied corticosteroids into the bloodstream, especially when these medications are potent, applied in large quantities too frequently, or used inappropriately under a diaper or other areas.

As such there may be a risk that topical steroids could slow a child's growth. However, it should be noted that the exact cause of growth impairment for children with chronic eczema is unclear, and there are conflicting studies on the topic. Some researchers have suggested routine monitoring of children who suffer from both severe atopic eczema and asthma and who also use corticosteroids. Another theory is that chronic stress and sleep disturbances caused by eczema may alter a child's growth hormone cycle. This could also be exacerbated by a poor or restricted diet or poor absorption of nutrition.

## GROWING CONCERNS WITHIN THE ECZEMA COMMUNITY

The growing awareness of the potential dangers of topical steroid overuse, and the horrific symptoms that some have experienced, ultimately led to the formation of the International Topical Steroid Addiction Network (ITSAN). The organization, which refers to this condition as red skin syndrome (RSS), offers online resources and information about the condition. Before ITSAN was founded in 2009, the condition was not well known, and little was being said about it. But since then, advocates such as Banos have become more vocal about TSW, and many have taken to social media and blogs to share firsthand accounts of their experiences.

The National Eczema Association (NEA) has also taken note of these increasing concerns within the eczema community. It responded by forming a task force of dermatologists to look more closely at this issue. The Scientific Advisory Committee Task Force—which Lio is part of—conducted a systematic review of topical corticosteroid withdrawal/addiction. The resulting article, published in the *Journal of the American Academy of Dermatology* in 2015, found that TSW was reported mostly on the face and genital area and that more women seemed to be affected. The review concluded that topical corticosteroid withdrawal is likely a distinct clinical adverse effect from misusing this topical medicine: "Patients and providers should be aware of its clinical presentations."

## HOW PREVALENT IS TSW?

TSW is sometimes described in medical literature as an emerging diagnosis. Because the medical world has yet to adopt standards for diagnosing TSW, it can be difficult to identify properly. Not only that, but often TSW is self-diagnosed by a patient rather than officially diagnosed by a physician, notes Lio.

TSW appears to affect women more than men. This may be because women tend to be more prone to allergic contact dermatitis, which may be the main diagnosis that leads to topical steroid use to begin with. Women are at higher risk for developing contact dermatitis because they tend to use more cosmetic products, Lio explains.

However, we don't have a good sense of how common or widespread this condition is. It's believed to be fairly rare, but it's hard to say based on the limited data currently available. The fact that it's likely rare may contribute to dermatologists' reluctance to address it.

"Most dermatologists I know who have been practicing for more than a decade, sometimes several decades, have not seen this either at all or much at all. Or at least they have not identified it as TSW," says Lio.

Sometimes it's hard to know whether a new condition or disease is truly a new entity or a variation of some other established condition, he notes.

# TOPICAL STEROID ALLERGY

One concern is that some TSW cases may actually be connected to other documented reactions to topical steroids. Topical steroids are known to cause conditions such as steroid-induced rosacea-like dermatitis, steroid-induced acne, and topical corticosteroid-damaged face. These conditions happen in people with high levels of corticosteroids, and in some cases, they can be attributed to overuse of topical steroids. These conditions may look similar to TSW, Silverberg notes.

Another documented condition that may be similar—or mistaken for—TSW is topical steroid allergy. Topical steroid allergy, or topical corticosteroid sensitivity, affects people who have a contact allergy or sensitivity to the inactive components (known as the vehicle) of a topical steroid. People who have a chronic skin condition and use multiple prescriptions (including over-the-counter topical steroids) are at higher risk of developing these allergies.

Topical steroid allergy was first reported many decades ago, and Silverberg believes that at least some of the cases thought to be TSW are actually caused by a topical steroid allergy. "It's a well-established phenomenon in the world of contact dermatitis that patients can pick up allergies over their lifetime to many different ingredients that they're using to treat their skin, whether it's prescription or over the counter," Silverberg says.

If you have an allergy or sensitivity to a topical corticosteroid, it can cause contact dermatitis, which can in turn cause severe skin eruptions and flares. The risk factors for developing topical steroid allergy include long-term, frequent application of topical steroids. But an allergy to topical steroids is particularly difficult to diagnose because the symptoms may be masked by the anti-inflammatory action of the corticosteroid itself. Also, the symptoms of contact dermatitis from topical steroids may be mixed with those of the underlying skin disease, such as eczema. So it's difficult to tell what symptoms are being caused by a reaction to topical corticosteroids and what might be an underlying acute eczema flare.

A topical steroid allergy may be diagnosed through a skin patch test, explains Silverberg. "You might actually be allergic to a preservative in the steroids. You may be missing a completely different diagnosis that could lend itself to avoidance and prevention of disease flares," he says.

However, this isn't to say that topical allergies are behind all the cases of TSW. There are situations where topical steroids are overused, and this can result in a host of side effects, Silverberg notes.

## TOPICAL STEROID PHOBIA

Part of the problem is that TSW itself hasn't been well defined, and it's still unclear how prevalent these cases are. For one, there is still no consensus in the medical world on the criteria used to diagnose TSW, notes Lio. "The hard part about topical steroid withdrawal is that there may be differing susceptibilities to it, so sometimes what seems safe for one patient may not be safe for another," he explains.

The heightened awareness of TSW has created apprehension among some patients. Some patients express a desire to avoid using topical steroids; some decline prescriptions or don't adhere to the regimen for medication usage, instead using far less than was prescribed.

Some recent medical journal articles refer to this as "topical corticosteroid phobia." In one study, published in *JAMA Dermatology* in October 2017, the authors conducted a search through medical literature from 1946 to 2016 to gain a better understanding of these concerns and fears. They found that a "phobia" or aversion to using topical steroids was fairly common among patients. Not surprisingly, those who had this fear were much more likely to not adhere to the treatment regimen. The study's authors noted that nonadherence was likely a contributing factor to poor patient outcomes.

Ultimately, patients need to be comfortable with their treatment. Like most things when it comes to eczema, there is no one-size-fits-all treatment, notes Silverberg.

"Topical steroid withdrawal is a very sensitive topic. It evokes a lot of emotions out of a lot of people," Silverberg says. "By and large, the overwhelming majority of patients tolerate topical steroids. But it's a conversation to be had with your clinician and something that (physicians) have to keep in mind when we're setting treatment, so we can share the decision making."

## HOW DO YOU TREAT TSW?

Many people going through TSW grapple with the symptoms of withdrawal, and many are desperate to find ways to manage these severe symptoms and effective treatments that can help them through this process. The first step in treating topical steroid addiction is to stop all use of steroids, including topical, inhaled, and systemic, provided that this can be done safely. Beyond that, there aren't any definitive guidelines. Those going through the process often turn to alternative treatments and natural remedies in hopes of finding something to help them detox and heal from topical steroids.

But doctors are also beginning to look at ways to help patients through this process. There are a number of medical treatments and therapies that are being tried out to support patients going through TSW, explains Lio in a 2019 *Practical Dermatology* journal article. The process of going through withdrawal can be complicated because the underlying eczema may also flare up in conjunction with discontinuing topical steroids, and because it's hard to tell an eczema flare from TSW symptoms. "Once TSW has been identified, the first step is discontinuation of all steroids (topical, inhaled, and systemic) if not already done so, and provided that they can be stopped safely," Lio writes. Unfortunately, few medical guidelines exist beyond this step, but there are many different therapeutic options that may help treat withdrawal symptoms.

Some doctors have treated symptoms of TSW by using a gradual steroid taper, Lio writes in the journal article. A taper is used to slowly wean the person off of all oral or topical steroids the person may be using. An oral steroid taper would gradually reduce the dosage of oral steroids a patient may be taking, along with gradually reducing topical steroids being used on the body, until the person is no longer using steroids of any form. The idea is that if someone abruptly stopped steroids, they could end up in a severe rebound flare, explains Lio. A steroid taper could in theory help ease symptoms of TSW and lead to a better treatment result for the patient. But Lio hasn't used this approach with his own patients.

"My personal approach is to try to totally avoid steroids in these folks because I don't know if more steroids could simply prolong the TSW," Lio explains in an email interview. "Most of my patients have also wanted to totally avoid them, so I don't have any experience with using them in this way."

If you wish to avoid steroids altogether, other conventional medical therapies can be used for managing TSW symptoms, including nonsteroidal oral or topical medications, explains Lio. There are a range of antibiotics, antihistamines, and topical and oral drugs that aren't steroids but can reduce inflammation in the skin.

Some conventional therapies that some doctors use to manage TSW symptoms while a patient goes off topical steroids include the following:

**Tetracycline**—This is an antibiotic that fights infection caused by bacteria.

**Calcineurin Inhibitors**—This is a class of drugs that includes topical tacrolimus (Protopic) and pimecrolimus (Elidel) and oral cyclosporine. These drugs have an immunosuppressive effect, meaning they act on the immune system to reduce skin inflammation. They block a chemical called calcineurin, which is an enzyme that activates T cells in the immune system.

**Phototherapy**—Sometimes called light therapy, this a non-pharmacological treatment that involves using narrow-band ultraviolet light, which is considered the "best part" of sunlight. This therapy usually involves multiple weekly visits to a doctor's office to use a special machine, which may look similar to a tanning booth. Varying forms of phototherapy have long been used to treat eczema and other skin disorders.

**Dupilumab (Dupixent)**—This is a relatively new drug that received US Food and Drug Administration (FDA) approval in 2017. Administered by injection, it's the first biologic approved for moderate to severe chronic eczema. It has been called a breakthrough drug because it's the first long-term, systemic drug to treat chronic eczema. Dupilumab has shown promise as a novel therapy to help a patient recover from TSW.

## DUPILUMAB: A NOVEL THERAPY THAT MAY PROVE EFFECTIVE FOR TSW

Lio was among a group of doctors who did a retrospective chart review on a handful of cases where patients used dupilumab while going through TSW. The small case study looked at five people (three women and two men), most of whom had been using mid-to-high-potency topical steroids and had severe symptoms of TSW. All the patients had tried other conventional treatments, such as calcineurin inhibitors, which were all unsuccessful. After using dupilumab for a period of time, usually several months, all of them saw improvement in their eczema and TSW symptoms.

More studies are needed to determine how effective this would be with a larger group of people, notes Lio. But this review shows that dupilumab may be a valuable way to help patients get through the withdrawal symptoms.

# CHAPTER 10

# TREATING ECZEMA IN SKIN OF COLOR

Historically, dermatologists have largely focused on treating patients from the perspective of how skin conditions and treatments affect patients with fairer skin tones. But as we all know, our world is made up of a beautiful palette of skin colors and tones. While medications and treatments for eczema have been found to work similarly for everyone, regardless of race or ethnicity, what sometimes gets missed are the specific challenges or concerns that come with treating patients whose skin tones range across the spectrum.

In dermatology, the term "skin of color" is used to describe the darker skin of individuals from a broad and diverse range of racial and ethnic groups. Skin of color can pose some unique challenges when it comes to diagnosing and treating atopic dermatitis. Eczema can sometimes look and behave a little differently depending on the color and tone of the skin, and research shows that certain groups are more at risk of developing eczema, says Dr. Andrew Alexis, director of the Skin of Color Center at Mount Sinai West in New York. He is also the chair of the Department of Dermatology at Mount Sinai West and professor of dermatology at the Icahn School of Medicine at Mount Sinai. Alexis was interviewed by phone for this book.

The Skin of Color Center was founded 20 years ago to address distinctions in skin types and identify ways that dermatologists can better diagnose and treat skin conditions in people with skin of color. Alexis is actively involved in advancing patient care, research, and education pertaining to dermatologic disorders that are prevalent in ethnic skin.

The Skin of Color Center works to advance the following goals, Alexis says:

- Advancing patient care for various dermatologic conditions that are prevalent among people of color

- Advancing research into conditions that disproportionately affect patients of color and where there are many unmet therapeutic needs

- Diagnosing and treating skin conditions more common to, or of particular concern to people of color, including African Americans, Asians, and Latinos

- Educating both the medical/dermatological community and the general community about skin diseases that affect skin, hair, and nail conditions in patients of color

## ECZEMA AFFECTS MORE PEOPLE OF COLOR

Eczema affects people from all different backgrounds, races, and ethnicities, but it appears to be more prevalent in African Americans, Alexis notes. The reasons for this are not clear, but it is likely due to a combination of factors. Specifically, research has found that eczema seems to be more prevalent in children of African ancestry. According to the Centers for Disease Control and Prevention (CDC), the prevalence of eczema increased among children of all races and ethnicities between 2000 and

2010. According to the CDC's data, African American children had the greatest increase in diagnoses. The CDC reports that eczema affects around 11 percent of children overall.

The National Eczema Association (NEA) reports that the racial and ethnic breakdown of children in the US with eczema includes the following:

- 20.2 percent of African American children
- 13 percent of Asian children
- 13 percent of Native American children
- 12.1 percent of white children
- 10.7 percent of Hispanic children

However, those statistics tend to change as people age. According to NEA, the racial and ethnic breakdown of adults with eczema includes the following:

- 7.7 percent of African American adults
- 9.1 percent of Asian adults
- 7.8 percent of Native American adults
- 10.5 percent of white adults
- 10.8 percent of Hispanic adults

Some studies have found that African Americans may experience more significant or severe symptoms from the disease. One study, published in 2018 in the *Annals of Allergy, Asthma & Immunology*, found that African Americans faced greater treatment challenges than patients of European ancestry. Another study, published in 2017 in the *Journal of the American Academy of Dermatology*, found that minority children were less likely to see a physician for treatment and more likely to have asthma along with eczema.

# WHY IS ECZEMA MORE COMMON IN CERTAIN ETHNIC GROUPS?

We aren't sure why people of African ancestry are more prone to eczema, but researchers believe that genetic and environmental factors may influence a person's risk of developing eczema. Typically, people with a family history of eczema or other atopic diseases, such as food allergies, asthma, or hay fever, are more likely to have the condition.

We also know that certain genetic mutations that affect the skin barrier cells and skin immune cells are inherited. Researchers also believe that these mutations tend to occur more often in some ethnic groups than in others, which may help explain differences in the frequency and severity of eczema between whites, African Americans, Asians, Hispanics, and others.

In addition, people who live in an urban setting or are exposed to certain environmental allergens, such as dust and mold, are at greater risk of developing atopic dermatitis.

# ECZEMA ERYTHEMA AND LESIONS IN SKIN OF COLOR

Some aspects of eczema may look different in people with darker skin tones, and such patients may have different reaction patterns, explains Alexis. One of the challenges of diagnosing eczema in patients with skin of color is the ability to detect erythema, or redness of the skin, because its appearance can vary according to skin tone, explains Alexis.

"When eczema presents clinically, there can be challenges in making the diagnosis or accurately assessing the severity, for one, because the redness or erythema can be masked or altered by the background pigment of the skin," says Alexis. Dermatologists are often taught to identify eczema based on certain clinical features, such as bright red "plaques" or patches of inflamed skin. But when it comes to darker skin types, that redness may take on different shades, such as purple or violet. Erythema can also look gray-brown, red-brown, or very dark brown. It may resemble increased pigment, so it can be confused with hyperpigmentation, Alexis notes.

"So, the eye has to be calibrated and trained to be able to detect the nuances of what redness looks like in the background of melanin-rich pigmented skin," he explains.

These differences in appearance sometimes make it hard to perceive how severe a case of eczema may be. This is why it's important for you to let your doctor or dermatologist know what your skin looks like when it's flaring. If you know that it doesn't turn red but rather more purple or darker brown, you need to communicate that to your doctor during your appointment, Alexis says.

## COMMON PRESENTATIONS OF ECZEMA MAY BE DIFFERENT

Another diagnostic challenge is that some eczema lesions may look different in patients with skin of color. This is called the morphology of eczema and refers to the common ways the disease presents, or appears.

For example, there is a tendency for people with skin of color to have a follicular presentation of eczema, which is a collection of small, itchy bumps that are between one and three millimeters in size, Alexis notes. These bumps, or papules, have no fluid or pus in them, and they may or may not occur with other typical eczema symptoms.

Follicular eczema commonly develops on the torso, arms, and legs. If the eczema is severely itchy, the papules may be scratched open, so the skin may be covered in small scabs, which can also obscure its appearance. And while these bumps may look red in fairer skin tones, they may look dark brown, red-brown, or purplish in color against a darker skin tone.

Another clinical variation that can occur in people of color with eczema is called a lichenoid variant. This variation of eczema presents with small, purplish bumps that often develop in the extensor surfaces of the body, which include the knees and the elbows.

"It can sometimes be a challenge to differentiate a lichenoid variant from another condition that also presents purplish bumps, called lichen planus, which is another scaly, itchy disorder," Alexis says. Lichen planus is also characterized by an itchy, noninfectious rash on the arms and legs and may consist of small, many-sided, flat-topped pink or purple bumps. Some specialists believe that lichen planus is an autoimmune disease. "Lichenoid variant is still eczema, but it has features that mimic a completely different inflammatory, itchy disease," explains Alexis.

There may be some immune system variations between eczema patients of different populations that may also affect how eczema presents. For example, some East Asian patients may have a unique form of eczema that resembles psoriasis. Because it mimics some symptoms of psoriasis, it is called psoriasiform dermatitis. These variations in presentation may have to do with immunologic differences between patients, or how their immune systems respond differently to some aspects of the disease.

## SKIN DAMAGE FROM CHRONIC ITCHING

When patients have been dealing with chronic eczema for months or years, the constant itching and scratching may cause the skin to develop thicker, discolored plaques. This is called lichenification. It's crucial to get eczema under control as quickly as possible to avoid the type of long-term skin damage that can come from lichenification.

Patients with African ancestry also have a greater frequency of an eczema-associated condition called prurigo nodularis, in which hard, itchy, crusty lumps or nodules form on the skin. This condition can be intensely itchy and very hard to treat.

We're not sure why people with African ancestry might be more prone to developing prurigo nodularis and other eczematous skin conditions, but some emerging research suggests that certain populations, including African Americans, may have a tendency toward more severe pruritus, or itching, associated with their eczema, which can lead to long-term scratching and rubbing of the affected area.

What we do know is that eczema and the associated itching and scratching can cause damage to the skin if it's not properly controlled. If these itchy skin conditions persist for years, they can also leave behind pigmentary changes in the skin that persist even after the eczema is under control. This skin damage can involve increased pigment, which is called hyperpigmentation, or a loss of pigment, called depigmentation. The latter can occur when scratching causes permanent damage to the skin's pigment-forming cells, Alexis explains.

# SKIN-CARE REGIMENS
# FOR SKIN OF COLOR

Maintaining a good skin-care routine can help reduce eczema flares and keep eczema itch under control. This can in turn reduce the risk and severity of long-term pigmentary changes to the skin. As with any skin type, treating eczema in skin of color begins with maintaining the skin barrier through gentle cleansing and moisturizing and avoiding letting the skin get dried out. These steps are key to protecting the skin barrier and helping the skin repair itself.

Alexis recommends using gentle, moisturizing skin cleansers and body washes that won't dry the skin out. Even washing with water alone can remove natural moisturizing factors from the skin. And cleansing with traditional soap will strip away even more of these natural moisturizing factors and lipids, which will cause the skin to dry out faster. So it's crucial to avoid harsher soaps, which can contribute to the breakdown of the skin barrier, increasing dryness and inflammation in eczema-prone skin.

It's also important to avoid any products that might be irritating. Skin with eczema tends to be more sensitive, so it's best to avoid fragranced skin-care products. This also goes for natural remedies or products. Although some natural products may be helpful, they aren't necessarily risk free, Alexis notes. You can still have allergic reactions to natural remedies or products, such as tea tree oil or coconut oil. Alexis recommends being watchful of what products you use, whether they are natural or synthetic.

# SPECIAL CONCERNS WHEN CARING FOR SKIN OF COLOR

There may be some subtle differences in the stratum corneum, or the outermost layer of the skin, that make people of African ancestry more susceptible to dry skin. Some studies have found that people of African ancestry tend to have a lower amount of ceramide in their skin than people of European or Asian ancestry. Found in the upper layer of the skin, ceramide is a waxy lipid or fatty acid that is produced by the skin and helps it retain its moisture.

One Danish study conducted in 2010 looked at the ceramide content in the skin of patients with Asian, Danish, and African ancestry and found that those of African ancestry had the lowest content of lipids in the upper layer of skin. This lower lipid content may help explain why people of African ancestry are more prone to severe eczema, Alexis notes.

This is another reason why it's so important for people with skin of color who have eczema to avoid letting their skin get overly dry and to maintain moisturization of the skin. Alexis recommends replenishing the skin through liberal use of creams and moisturizers as soon as you finish bathing. He also stresses that it's important to control inflammation and reduce flares in a timely manner.

Maintaining the skin's moisture is the first step toward diminishing and controlling chronic cases of eczema and avoiding permanent skin damage or changes to skin pigmentation. If traditional therapies and skin-care regimens aren't working, it may be time to consider other systemic medications, Alexis notes.

# TOPICAL STEROIDS AND HYPOPIGMENTATION

The use of topical corticosteroids is an important and useful treatment for all eczema patients because it is one of the most effective ways to get an eczema flare under control, Alexis says. These topical medications help dermatologists manage and control eczema flares, and they are still more effective than other topical medications on the market. But corticosteroids are best used as an intermittent, short-term treatment, and as just one part of an overall strategy to control long-term, active eczema. To reduce overall damage to the skin, it's crucial to come up with an effective long-term strategy to manage eczema.

It's particularly important that people with darker skin tones are aware that topical corticosteroids can cause pigmentary changes to the skin if used for too long, Alexis explains. Overuse or long-term use of topical steroids is associated with hypopigmentation, which is the temporary lightening of the skin, Alexis explains. Depigmentation and hypopigmentation are similar in that both conditions result in changes to pigmentation in the skin, but there are a few key distinctions. Hypopigmentation is the temporary reduction of skin color in an area, so the skin becomes lighter than the baseline skin color. Depigmentation is a permanent loss of pigment or color, Alexis explains. Depigmentation can result from chronic injury, such as scratching the skin for many years. Hypopigmentation can sometimes result from long-term use of potent topical steroids.

Hypopigmentation can be a significant and distressing issue for patients with darker skin tones. This potential side effect from topical steroids tends to be more striking and disfiguring in darker skin tones than in lighter ones, and it's far more noticeable, Alexis notes. The risk of hypopigmentation increases the more potent the topical steroid and the longer it's used.

"We still use corticosteroids, but these concerns speak to the importance of having the oversight of a dermatologist or other medical expert in managing your eczema," Alexis says. "It's important to monitor the strength of the steroids, the amount that is used, and the duration for which it's used."

One example of a strategy to consider would be using a corticosteroid for two weeks and then tapering down and transitioning to non-corticosteroid therapies for a more extended period of time. The goal is to keep eczema managed, so that topical steroids are only needed occasionally, during a flare-up, while other therapies are used more frequently to keep skin in check. An approach such as this can help mitigate the risk of hypopigmentation and the thinning of the skin, Alexis explains.

Aggressively treating eczema and controlling the itch will also reduce the risk and severity of any long-term pigment changes, Alexis says. This is why it's important to avoid undertreating eczema, but also to make sure all treatments are being used as safely and effectively as possible, he explains.

## NON-CORTICOSTEROID THERAPIES FOR LONG-TERM MANAGEMENT

There is a growing list of non-corticosteroid treatments that are important additions to the arsenal of eczema-treatment therapies. Topical corticosteroids aren't ideal for long-term management. They are best used in the short term to gain control over flare-ups. But once eczema is under control, non-corticosteroids can be swapped in to help maintain longer-term control over the disease, explains Alexis.

"Because eczema is a chronic-relapsing condition, we benefit from therapies that can be used continuously over the long-term," he says.

Non-corticosteroids include the following:

• Calcineurin inhibitors, such as Protopic and Elidel

• Topical PDE4 inhibitors, such as crisaborole (Eucrisa)

• Dupilumab (Dupixent), the first injectable biologic medicine to offer continuous treatment of moderate to severe eczema

Studies have found no adverse reactions when using these therapies in skin of color.

In addition, a number of new therapies are going through development and clinical trials and should become available in the coming months and years.

"There is a whole pipeline of new therapies, such as JAK inhibitors, oral and topical therapies," Alexis explains. "These will help us manage this long-term disorder with therapies that aren't associated with the side effects of steroids." Some of these exciting new therapies are discussed further in Chapter 12.

Corticosteroids still have their place in the lineup of treatments, and they are very safe and effective for short-term and intermittent use, Alexis notes. "But what has been missing in the past is non-corticosteroid agents that we could use for long-term control with minimal risk."

# CHAPTER 11

# ECZEMA'S IMPACT ON MENTAL HEALTH AND OVERALL WELL-BEING

The impacts of eczema go much deeper than the skin. We are beginning to realize that this disease can have startling impacts on a person's physical, mental, and social well-being. Researchers have begun to look beyond the skin's surface, and the resulting studies are shedding more light on the far-reaching effects this disease can have, not just on those who are contending with the disease, but also their family members and those who help care for them.

Eczema has also been shown to directly and deeply affect a person's overall health in ways we didn't fully realize until recently. People with chronic eczema are more likely to engage in unhealthy behaviors, such as drinking and smoking, while also being less likely to exercise. And people with eczema are more likely to suffer from cardiovascular problems or autoimmune conditions, among other health issues, says professor of dermatology Dr. Jonathan Silverberg.

Recent studies have also found that people with eczema are at higher risk for developing more than one condition or chronic disease, known as comorbidities. As more research is being conducted in this area, we are gaining a better understanding of how these conditions may be interconnected. The following are some of the comorbidities of eczema:

- Depression
- Anxiety
- Attention deficit hyperactivity disorder
- Suicidal ideation/suicidal thoughts
- Obesity
- High blood pressure
- Heart disease
- Diabetes
- Infection
- Allergic conditions such as food allergies, asthma, and hay fever

Some of these conditions, such as allergies, have long been known to occur alongside eczema. It is also well established that people with eczema are more prone to bacterial infections of the skin, such as staph infections, impetigo, and cellulitis. But a number of other comorbidities have gone relatively unnoticed.

One the most significant and overlooked impacts is on mental health. If you have chronic eczema, you are much more likely to also grapple with anxiety and depression. Not only that, but people with eczema are more likely to harbor suicidal thoughts than those without the condition. Studies have also found that family members are often impacted. Parents and caregivers of those who have chronic eczema often suffer from anxiety and depression as well.

# HOW DOES ECZEMA IMPACT PEOPLE?

Understanding the broader impacts of eczema requires taking a closer look at this disease's symptoms and having more awareness of how the disease affects daily life. As we've discussed, eczema's common symptoms include inflamed, red skin; swelling, oozing, and crusting; rough and leathery skin; and of course, horribly itchy skin.

The appearance of eczema—the way it looks on your skin—often has a social impact on those who contend with this disease. That rashy, oozy skin can cause feelings of embarrassment and be a source of distress on its own. If your eczema is noticeable in places on the body that can't be covered up, such as your face or hands, you may feel like others are constantly making judgments about how you look and perhaps assuming that your rash is contagious.

The International Study of Life with Atopic Eczema—the first large-scale study to assess the effects of eczema on the lives of patients and society—found that eczema has major impacts on confidence and self-esteem. Children with eczema often find they are targets of bullying or teasing by other children, with 39 percent of children between 8 and 17 years old reporting that they were teased or bullied because of eczema. The 2006 study also found that over half of parents interviewed reported that they themselves limited interactions between their children and family and friends so that they wouldn't have to engage in discussion about their child's skin.

Adults with eczema may feel like others are scrutinizing their appearance, which can cause them to want to hide their skin or avoid social situations. The International Study of Life with

Atopic Eczema found that 43 percent of people with eczema felt concerned about being seen in public and 42 percent reported feeling awkward about a partner touching or seeing their body during a flare. More than half reported that they were unhappy or depressed, and 36 percent said eczema affects their self-confidence. Sadly, it seems that living daily life with eczema can leave you feeling socially stigmatized and detached from others.

## ITCHINESS, SKIN PAIN, AND SLEEP DISTURBANCES

Beyond the emotional distress of eczema, it's the relentless itch that patients often rank as the most debilitating and burdensome symptom they must deal with. One study found that 91 percent of survey respondents reported they itched daily, and more than 70 percent reported having a severe or unbearable itch within the last two weeks. In addition to this constant itchiness, there is another symptom that often gets overlooked: skin pain.

Many people with eczema also deal with skin pain, which may be associated with itchy skin and scratching, but skin pain isn't widely recognized or addressed by doctors, Silverberg says. One study found that more than half of people with eczema surveyed reported having pain associated with the skin condition. And of those who reported pain, nearly 14 percent said their pain levels were severe or very severe and 72 percent said they believed the pain was from itching and scratching. Yet most physicians don't recognize skin pain as a symptom of eczema—it simply isn't on their radar, Silverberg notes.

As a consequence of itching and pain, people with eczema often deal with chronic sleep disturbances. The chronic itchiness and pain of eczema makes it hard to fall asleep and stay asleep, resulting in shorter sleep durations. Thus, it's harder to wake up in the morning and feel ready to meet the challenges of the day.

People with eczema are often sleep deprived and exhausted, which undoubtedly contributes to a poorer quality of life. Some studies have found that people with eczema who experience chronic sleep disturbances also deal with memory impairment and difficulty functioning at work or school. This can also lead to mood swings and behavioral problems.

The reality is that if you are wrestling with itchy, painful skin, you're likely not sleeping well at night. If you aren't able to sleep well, it's difficult to focus and be productive at work or concentrate at school. Not to mention that the persistent itch, day and night, is itself a continual distraction, on top of the exhaustion you're feeling from not getting enough sleep.

## THE CONNECTION BETWEEN ECZEMA AND INATTENTIVENESS

Children with eczema may also have a higher chance of being diagnosed with attention deficit hyperactivity disorder (ADHD). A growing body of research is showing a link between eczema and symptoms of ADHD, especially when the eczema is severe.

One theory is that the chronic itchiness and sleep disturbances associated with eczema may, in part, explain why children with eczema have higher rates of ADHD. According to one study coauthored by Silverberg and published in 2016, children with severe eczema and chronic sleep disturbance had an increased risk of ADHD. That study found that children with severe eczema get less than three nights of adequate sleep per week, whereas children with mild to moderate eczema get adequate sleep four or more nights a week. Those children with severe eczema who were getting only a few nights of adequate sleep per week had a much higher risk of ADHD.

In addition, the study found that children were at increased risk of developing ADHD if they had eczema and asthma or if they had eczema and also dealt with headaches, obesity, or anemia. Another finding was that adults with eczema were at increased risk of having ADHD, and the risk was even higher for adults who also had a history of asthma, headaches, or insomnia.

## ANXIETY AND STRESS AS SYMPTOMS OF ECZEMA

Studies on eczema and quality of life clearly show how big an impact this skin condition has on mental health. According to a 2019 study published in the *British Journal of Dermatology* and coauthored by Silverberg, half of all adults with chronic eczema experience anxiety or depression. The findings were based on a survey of 2,893 US adults as part of a study aimed at understanding the burden of eczema in adults, Silverberg explains.

Among the study's impactful findings: the more severe the case of eczema, the more likely the patient was to also have symptoms of anxiety and depression. One startling revelation was that virtually all patients with severe eczema had symptoms of depression and anxiety. It's rare in research to have a finding that affects 100 percent of patients in a category.

It's especially surprising that anxiety and depression symptoms would be found to be so common in any group of people, Silverberg notes. Approximately 7 percent of adults say they have eczema, and of those, 40 percent say they have moderate to severe forms of eczema, according to a 2018 survey on the prevalence of eczema in US adults. That means that roughly 6.6 million adults in the US have chronic, potentially life-disrupting eczema and are at higher risk of having anxiety and depression; they are also more likely to see impacts in other areas of their overall health. On the whole, anxiety disorders are estimated to affect about 18 percent of the general population.

Health-care providers have long understood that there is a connection between the mind and the skin, and they have long acknowledged an association between skin conditions such as eczema and secondary psychiatric disorders. Often, stress and anxiety were (and are still) believed to be exacerbating factors in triggering a flare.

When patients with a particularly difficult case of eczema don't respond to treatment, physicians have been advised to ask the patient if stress, in either their personal or their work life, might be contributing to their skin disorder. The idea is that the impact of those stressors might be contributing to flares. But if Silverberg's research is any indication, doctors should also consider whether eczema itself is potentially a root cause of some patients' mental health issues. Doctors are now understanding that moderate to severe eczema may be causing anxiety, depression, and inattentiveness for many patients.

## CONTROLLING ECZEMA CAN IMPROVE MENTAL HEALTH

Living with eczema can be like living on a rollercoaster; each day you're uncertain what unexpected concern you might wake up to when you examine your skin. Dealing with this alone can be a source of constant anxiety. But what people may not realize is that eczema takes an emotional and mental toll that often goes unseen.

Eczema can have a direct impact on mental health, Silverberg says. It's becoming clear that mental health symptoms are just as much a problem as itch or skin pain. This may sound like a surprising theory to some, but Silverberg points to a mountain of research and conclusive data as well as multiple firsthand observations.

One example that crystallized this for researchers was the feedback they got from patients during clinical trials for dupilumab, in which Silverberg was heavily involved. During those clinic trials, doctors noticed that among eczema patients with anxiety and depression, when their skin cleared during treatment with dupilumab, their anxiety and depression tended to improve as well. Dupilumab doesn't have any effect as an antidepressant, but once patients successfully got their eczema under control, improvements in their mental health seemed to naturally follow. So, for many people, improving or eliminating the most troublesome and burdensome symptoms of eczema has an impact far beyond just clearing their skin.

"When you talk to patients and when you see how debilitating eczema can be for them and the amazing impact one can have on their lives when you get them feeling better, it's truly unbelievable," says Silverberg.

This is why it's so important to look at ways to treat eczema as a condition that requires a multidisciplinary approach, especially when it comes to aspects and concerns that impact mental health, such as depression, anxiety, and sleep disturbances. Silverberg says that the goal should be to take a holistic approach to treating the whole patient instead of just focusing on the skin.

# DEPRESSION IN PARENTS

The impact on mental health often goes beyond the patient. Another aspect that is often overlooked is the effect that a young child's eczema diagnosis can have on family members who are helping care for the child. The weight of this diagnosis and the responsibility of being constantly vigilant in managing the child's condition—which also entails sorting through treatment options and weighing potential benefits and adverse effects—can leave parents and caregivers grappling with their own anxiety, emotional distress, and insomnia.

It has also been noted that eczema may impact the mother-child attachment and bonding that happens early on in life. This important attachment between mother and child is harder to achieve when the mother is contending with a baby who is constantly fussy and itchy, not sleeping well, and unable to be soothed. A 2016 study found that mothers with infants who had eczema were more likely to describe themselves as feeling depressed, hopeless, anxious, and overprotective.

And these feelings of depression and anxiety may affect the whole family of a child dealing with chronic eczema. A 2019 study found that a majority of family members and caregivers of children with chronic eczema suffer from anxiety and depression. The study was conducted through the PHI University Clinic of Dermatology in Skopje, Republic of North Macedonia. Researchers assessed the impact of an atopic dermatitis diagnosis on the families of 35 children between the ages of one and six. They evaluated 83 family members and caregivers and found that all of them reported at least mild anxiety, with some showing moderate anxiety. Almost three in four were also found to have depression.

According to the study's findings, depression and anxiety scores were associated with the persistence and longevity of atopic dermatitis. Parents also faced the need to be constantly vigilant about their child's treatment regimen, closely monitoring everything from what clothes they wear to what foods they eat and what activities they are involved in, as these can all be possible triggers for eczema.

## SUICIDAL THOUGHTS

People who deal with the endless itching, skin-disfiguring lesions, weeping skin, and rashes of eczema are not just at a great risk for developing depression; the condition can also leave some more vulnerable to suicidal thoughts and possibly suicide attempts. A 2019 study out of the University of Southern California looked at the links between eczema and suicidal thoughts. The researchers sifted through 15 studies involving nearly 5 million people and over 300,000 eczema patients. According to the results of the meta-analysis, eczema patients were 44 percent more likely to exhibit suicidal ideation (having thoughts of or planning suicide), and 36 percent more likely to attempt suicide, than people without the condition.

The study observed that patients with uncontrolled eczema often had to deal with debilitating itching, burning, and skin pain as well as lack of sleep caused by these symptoms. The burden of these symptoms, coupled with chronic sleep loss and exhaustion, was shown to increase thoughts of suicide in patients with eczema. "By addressing the physical burden, psychosocial burden, and chronic inflammatory state of eczema, we can work toward reducing suicidality in patients with AD," the study's authors noted.

The data on individuals who took their own life was limited and showed inconsistent results. But the analysis makes it clear that the mental burden of eczema may have grave and dire ramifications. These and other study findings may spur dermatologists and other health-care providers to implement patient screenings or use questionnaires to gauge the risk levels and warning signs in patients who are dealing with these chronic symptoms.

## POOR HEALTH HABITS

People with eczema are also more likely to engage in poor health habits or riskier behaviors, and these may also impact overall health and contribute to a person's likelihood of developing some of these comorbidities. And yet smoking, or being around someone who smokes, can have particularly adverse effects if you have eczema, Silverberg notes. Smoke may be an irritant and could either trigger or worsen a flare.

People with eczema are also more likely to drink alcohol and to have higher consumption rates of alcohol. In addition, studies have found that adults with eczema have higher rates of smoking, and started smoking significantly younger than those without eczema. Meanwhile, they are less likely to engage in vigorous daily activity, and they have lower levels of being physically active than those who don't have eczema, which may be in part because sweating can aggravate eczema. This in turn is linked to another factor with broad health implications: if you're not exercising, you're more likely to be overweight.

# IMPACTS ON THE IMMUNE SYSTEM AND AUTOIMMUNE DISORDERS

Atopic dermatitis is an immunological disease, which means it involves the immune system: eczema causes the immune system to produce inflammation, which erupts on the skin. But there is ongoing debate as to whether eczema should be considered an autoimmune disorder, where a patient's immune system mistakenly attacks the body. Eczema is broadly categorized as an atopic disease, or allergic disease, which means it causes a heightened immune response when immune cells come into contact with certain allergens. It also appears eczema's impact on the immune system may put patients at risk for internal infections, including those of the upper respiratory tract and urinary tract.

Researchers have begun to recognize that there may be an association between autoimmune diseases and eczema. In a cross-sectional study of hospitalized adults and children in the US, patients with eczema were found to have higher rates of various autoimmune disorders—including those affecting the skin and the endocrine, gastrointestinal, hematologic, and musculoskeletal systems—than patients without eczema.

Recent cross-sectional studies of Danish and German populations have suggested an association between eczema and autoimmune conditions, such as alopecia areata, vitiligo, rheumatoid arthritis, Crohn's disease, and ulcerative colitis. A US-based study, published in 2019 in the *Journal of the American Academy of Dermatology*, confirms these results. The study found that in particular, eczema was associated with 18 of 32 autoimmune disorders in adults, and 13 of 24 autoimmune disorders in children, including disorders of the skin and the endocrine, gastrointestinal, hematologic, and musculoskeletal systems. However, the precise mechanisms of association between eczema and autoimmune disorders remain unknown.

This study used a representative cross-sectional sample of approximately 20 percent of US hospitalizations—a total of more than 87 million patients, including 9,290 adults and 10,196 children with eczema. The patients with eczema were analyzed and compared with patients without eczema. Adults and children with eczema were more likely to be male, nonwhite, and have asthma than patients without eczema. Children hospitalized with eczema were also more likely to have hay fever.

# LONG-TERM IMPACTS

Patients with long-lasting eczema are at high risk for developing significant health conditions during their lifetimes. This includes being prone to cardiovascular problems such as heart disease, high blood pressure, high cholesterol, and stroke. They also have higher odds of developing diabetes or being diagnosed as prediabetic during their lifetime.

The link between eczema and cardiovascular disease was explored in a study published in the *Journal of Allergy and Clinical Immunology* in 2019. In that study, researchers from the UK, Canada, Denmark, and the US pooled individual study findings together in a meta-analysis. The authors reviewed 19 population-based, observational studies that looked at the link between atopic eczema and cardiovascular diseases, including angina, heart attack, heart failure, and stroke. They also looked at whether increasing eczema severity had any impact on the risk of cardiovascular disease.

The study found that the risk of developing cardiovascular disease was 15 percent greater for people with moderate atopic eczema than for those with mild atopic eczema, and for people with severe atopic eczema, the risk was 32 percent greater.

It's still unclear what is behind the link between eczema and cardiovascular health. Some of these conditions may develop as a result of eczema's cumulative effects on the body over the years, Silverberg notes. This should emphasize the importance of having a healthy lifestyle as well as having more aggressive therapies available to better manage eczema. For this reason, Silverberg says, treatment should focus on not only improving symptoms in the short term but also managing the condition in the long term.

## WHAT'S BEHIND THESE INCREASED RISKS?

Doctors and researchers are still trying to understand the links between eczema and many of these comorbidities. Could it all go back to the impact of dealing with the burden of these chronic symptoms, which then negatively influence health behaviors and impede healthy activities? These impacts could ultimately put someone with eczema more at risk for developing other diseases or conditions. Or could the mechanisms of the disease itself, such as its inflammatory nature, subsequently impact bodily systems and thereby increase risks for a range of health problems? Unfortunately, it's mostly conjecture at this point, and there's probably not one simple answer to these questions, Silverberg notes.

For one, there's no doubt that having uncontrolled moderate to severe eczema is a debilitating and depressing condition, and this will have impacts on your mental state, and all of this will affect your health behaviors. And this is especially true because the disease often strikes young people, at a time when they are developing lifelong health habits. So it's likely that having a chronic disease of this nature will drive poorer health behaviors, Silverberg says.

For instance, studies found that people with eczema tend to have higher levels of obesity and are more likely to have hypertension, to have diabetes or be considered prediabetic, and to have higher levels of cholesterol. Some of these conditions can be influenced by poor health behaviors.

But can eczema, as an inflammatory and immune-driven disease, have an impact on your health? Again, current research and studies haven't been able to decipher a clear answer, Silverberg says. What he does believe is that reining in the disease and keeping it under control will help patients lead healthier, happier lives. But this also comes down to taking a more holistic approach with patients and helping them attain a healthier lifestyle once their eczema is under control.

"I don't think it's realistic to say that if someone has become sedentary, and now that their eczema is under control, they're magically going to start going back to the gym again," Silverberg notes. "It's not enough to just medicate, but we really have to address the whole patient and work on encouraging them to go back to the gym, and encourage them to stop smoking. These are smart recommendations to be making in medicine anyway, because it will be so much better for long-term health."

## HOW TO LIVE A HAPPIER, HEALTHIER LIFE

What would happen if we did a better job of managing this disease early in life? Too often the standard of care is undertreatment, which means that patients are needlessly suffering, Silverberg says. Compounding this is that the disease is often trivialized by health-care providers. They may dismiss eczema as not being very severe, without really seeing the bigger impact the disease is having on a person's quality of life.

And this rankles Silverberg. He challenges others in the health-care profession to look at the bigger picture with patients. "When eczema is in its moderate to severe form and the patient hasn't slept in a year, or they haven't gone to school in six months, at what point do you wake up and realize it's not just eczema, it's a life-threatening disease and it's ruining people's lives?" Silverberg implores.

# CHAPTER 12

# THE ERA OF ECZEMA: NEW THERAPIES ON THE HORIZON

A wave of medical research and development in the past decade has helped usher in what dermatologists are calling the "Era of Eczema." After many decades of limited treatment options and a general lack of understanding about how and why eczema develops, a revolution in medical technology has given scientists a window into the underpinnings of eczema. In the world of dermatology, eczema is finally taking center stage.

Huge strides have been made in the last 15 years in terms of offering new therapies and treatments for chronic eczema. Some of the newer treatments to hit the market include topical calcineurin inhibitors, such as pimecrolimus and tacrolimus, which are a new class of anti-inflammatory drugs that don't contain steroids. They work by stopping a piece of the immune system from "switching on," thus preventing certain eczema symptoms, such as redness and itch. These were among the first drugs developed for eczema that are classified as immunomodulators, meaning they are intended to help regulate or normalize an aspect of the immune system that has gone awry.

In recent years, scientists have made a number of breakthroughs in understanding the mechanisms behind the causes of eczema, paving the way for the development of new therapies and treatments that target these underlying issues. Researchers have been able to pinpoint many of the processes that go wrong for people who have eczema, and this has shed light on how therapies can more effectively combat this condition.

## TARGETED THERAPIES

Expanding medical research and knowledge has allowed doctors to move away from just treating the symptoms on the surface of the skin, and to begin treating the underlying issues through targeted therapies—which are more precise in targeting the areas of the skin and immune system that aren't functioning normally. Targeted therapies are generally expected to be more effective than older forms of treatment and to have fewer adverse side effects, and they have high safety profiles.

Two such new drugs that have come on the market in recent years include crisaborole, a topical drug sold under the brand name Eucrisa, and dupilumab, an injectable drug sold under the brand name Dupixent. But a slew of other drugs is currently in development, and doctors say they are hopeful many of them will soon be headed for approval by the US Food and Drug Administration (FDA).

Hopefully many of these new therapies and drugs will soon be on the market, so patients will have more treatment options, says Silverberg.

"For decades now, patients with eczema have really not had a lot of hope, but there really is a great reason to have hope now, with so many new treatments being developed within dermatology,"

Silverberg says. "Now we refer to this as the decade of eczema. It's an exciting time and a time when you can really have hope that some really cool new options will be coming soon."

These targeted therapies are designed to address the issues that are causing the disease in the first place. Much of our new understanding about the mechanisms that cause eczema can be linked to major breakthroughs that researchers made in studying psoriasis, another chronic inflammatory skin disease. This new body of research has helped researchers reveal the complex interactions between environmental triggers, immune factors, and skin barrier dysfunction, which help explain how and why eczema develops.

However, doctors caution that the mainstay of eczema treatment remains the same: controlling the condition by maintaining the skin barrier and using topical medications, including topical corticosteroids. Maintaining the skin barrier often comes down to having a consistent skin-care regimen that focuses on hydrating and moisturizing your skin and preventing skin infections. Topical medications are meant to control and manage occasional flares.

But for patients with more severe cases of eczema that can't be controlled with traditional therapies, modern medicine has new options on the horizon that include injected, oral, and topical medications that target the eczema at the source of the problem.

## THE "INSIDE OUT" OR THE "OUTSIDE IN" THEORY?

There are two main theories that researchers have long been debating when it comes to understanding what causes eczema to manifest: the "inside out" theory and the "outside in" theory. The "outside in" theory is that an impaired skin barrier (cracked, dry skin) allows external antigens, or irritating agents from our environment, to penetrate into the skin. This causes skin irritation and inflammation, which then leads to eczema. In this theory, eczema is primarily caused by these outside factors.

The "inside out" theory is that a person who develops eczema has inflammation of the skin first, before their skin barrier becomes impaired, and this inflammation may, in fact, cause skin barrier dysfunction. This inflammation of the skin weakens the skin barrier by reducing the production of filaggrin, a protein in the top layer of the skin that is essential to the regulation of the skin's integrity.

Researchers now believe that the cause of eczema is a combination of these two theories. There is a complex interaction of both genetic and environmental factors that can result in the dysregulation of the immune system. However, researchers have also noticed that these patterns of reactions may be different in the early stages of skin inflammation—particularly in babies and young children who are just beginning to develop eczema— versus later on, among older children and adults.

## DECIPHERING THE UNDERLYING CAUSES OF ECZEMA

Scientists believe there is no one single cause of eczema, and there are many theories regarding the underlying mechanisms behind it. But in the last several decades, scientists have begun to better understand the complex causes behind eczema, and using this knowledge, they have been able to begin developing many new exciting and novel therapies that better target the mechanisms that cause eczema. Current research is focused on investigating the roles of the immune system, the skin structure, gene mutations, defects in the skin cells (also known keratinocytes), and the skin surface microbiome (the community of microorganisms that live on our skin), among other factors.

We understand that the skin barrier in a person with eczema doesn't function properly, which makes it easier for the skin to lose moisture. Our skin barrier is important because it is meant to keep environmental factors out, protect our insides, and keep moisture and water in. But skin barrier dysfunction means the skin becomes dry and cracked more easily. People with eczema have abnormalities in the skin barrier involving the lipids, or fats, that are between the cells in the upper part of the skin, known as the stratum corneum. This makes the skin more permeable, a condition that some people call "leaky skin." This is why dermatologists believe it's so important to help maintain the skin barrier by regularly moisturizing and hydrating the skin: doing so will help the skin repel those irritating agents and keep eczema from flaring.

Scientists theorize that skin barrier dysfunction is due to an inherited abnormality in the skin's filaggrin. Abnormal filaggrin is associated with early-onset, severe, and persistent atopic dermatitis.

Environmental factors also play a role in the development of eczema. If you are predisposed to eczema and you come into contact with environmental factors—something outside your body—that you are sensitive to, it can trigger a flare. These triggers might be something you are allergic to or something that is irritating to your system. A trigger can even be an overproduction on your skin of certain bacteria, such as Staphylococcus aureus, which is a common cause of skin infections.

Researchers also believe that people with eczema have abnormalities within certain immune cells in the skin. One such abnormality is a chronic overactivation of the Th2 immune cells (also called Type 2 helper T cells). It is believed that skin barrier dysfunction, along with environmental factors and dysregulation of immune system cells, can create a cascade effect where cells in the skin begin an immune reaction that causes Th2 cells to skew in an abnormal way. This abnormal skewing affects proteins, known as cytokines and chemokines, which can drive inflammation.

One area that scientists are looking at is the role of cytokines within the Th2 pathway. The immune cells use cytokines, a group of proteins that act as chemical messengers for the immune system and help regulate immune responses. Cytokines from one cell (in this case the Th2 immune cells) can affect the actions of other cells by binding to receptors on the surface of other cells.

In developing these new eczema drugs, researchers are looking at a particular type of cytokines, called interleukins, which are proteins that regulate immune and inflammatory responses. There are a number of different interleukins, and each plays a different role. For instance, interleukin 4 (IL-4) and interleukin 13 (IL-13) are related cytokines that regulate many aspects of allergic inflammation, which are believed to play an important role in causing an eczema flare.

## NEW THERAPIES ON THE MARKET

The last few years have seen the approval of two new therapies, both of which are considered "first-in-class" drugs, meaning they use new and unique mechanisms of action for treating a medical condition.

**Crisaborole (Eucrisa)**—This is the first nonsteroidal topical medication that is a phosphodiesterase 4 (PDE4) inhibitor, meaning it works to reduce the production of the enzyme phosphodiesterase. By inhibiting the production of PDE4, it reduces the production of cytokines, which drive inflammation. Crisaborole was approved by the FDA in 2016. This drug has been shown to be effective and safe for mild to moderate eczema in children two years and older and adults. However, a small percentage of patients report stinging and burning in the skin site where the medication has been applied. Additional phosphodiesterase inhibitors are in clinical trials and are expected to come online soon.

**Dupilumab (Dupixent)**—This is a first-of-its-kind biologic drug approved for either adolescents or adults as a systemic treatment for eczema. This medication has been hailed by many as a "miracle drug," in part because of its effectiveness and safety profile. Dupilumab is an IL-4 and IL-13 blockade. It targets the receptor for those cytokines and shuts down the inflammation driven by IL-4 and IL-13, which would have been driven by the skewing of the Th2 immune cell pathway (also called the Type 2 pathway). Dupilumab is administered by injection, usually every other week. The main side effects of this drug have been conjunctivitis, or inflammation of the eye, as well as reactions at the injection site.

In 2019 dupilumab was approved by the FDA to treat adolescents ages 12 to 17 with moderate to severe atopic dermatitis that can't be effectively controlled through other treatments. Clinical trials for using dupilumab to treat adolescents found that the drug significantly improved symptoms of chronic eczema and overall quality of life. It was also shown to be as effective and safe for adolescents as it is for adults.

Clinical trials are underway to evaluate dupilumab as a treatment for younger children. A phase 3 clinical trial is looking at using dupilumab in children from 6 to 11 years old with severe eczema. This is the first time a biologic medicine has been assessed in children under the age of 12. This study is examining the effectiveness of the drug when used along with topical corticosteroids. The results at 16 weeks found that 70 percent of patients who received dupilumab every four weeks and 67 percent of those who received the drug every two weeks achieved 75 percent or greater skin improvement; and 33 percent of patients who received dupilumab every four weeks and 30 percent of patients who received the drug every two weeks achieved clear or almost clear skin.

## NEW TREATMENTS IN THE PIPELINE

The treatment of eczema has become a rapidly evolving field with many new, cutting-edge therapies in the works, says Dr. Peter Lio, founding director of the Chicago Integrative Eczema Center.

These new treatments range from biologic agents, to anti-itch agents, to Janus kinase inhibitors (see page 202), many of which have shown great promise during clinical trials. There are also some exciting new topical treatments, some of which may offer intriguing options for patients who are interested in more natural approaches. Some of these may offer the best of both worlds, drawing from scientifically backed medicine and clinical effectiveness while utilizing forms traditionally thought of as being natural or alternative approaches.

# NEW ANTIBODIES

Two new biologic drugs that look promising for the treatment of eczema are lebrikizumab and tralokinumab. Both are human monoclonal antibodies, meaning they are antibodies that are made in a laboratory and engineered to neutralize certain pathogens, thus enhancing an immune system attack on those pathogens.

In this case, lebrikizumab and tralokinumab target the Type 2 pathway, the same arm of the immune system that dupilumab targets. However, instead of inhibiting both IL-4 and IL-13 cytokines, these antibodies just target IL-13. The cytokine IL-13 is believed to drive multiple aspects of eczema by promoting Type 2 inflammation. This inflammation can cause skin barrier dysfunction, itch, skin thickening, and infection. In theory, targeting just IL-13 might maximize efficacy and limit drug toxicity.

**Lebrikizumab**—This drug is administered by injection and works by binding with IL-13, preventing formation of a certain protein complex and a set of biologic signals that are linked with eczema. Lebrikizumab is being evaluated in two phase 3 clinical trials to confirm its safety and efficacy in adolescents and adults ages 12 years and older with moderate to severe eczema. The FDA has granted fast-track designation for lebrikizumab, which is meant to expedite review of a drug to treat serious conditions with an unmet medical need.

**Tralokinumab**—This is another drug that uses human monoclonal antibody, which neutralizes the IL-13 cytokine, a crucial driver of the Type 2 inflammation that plays a significant role in eczema. The drug has completed phase 3 clinical trials and was found to be safe and effective for treating adults with moderate to severe eczema. Overall, the adverse event rate between tralokinumab and the placebo was similar. It is expected to file for FDA approval.

## OTHER TARGETED THERAPIES

The Th2 pathway includes other cytokines and chemokines, some of which are considered good candidates for eczema drugs. These are some investigational therapies that are in development and that are looking at targeting other receptors.

**Nemolizumab**—This humanized antibody is administered by injection. Like lebrikizumab and tralokinumab, this drug works on the Type 2 pathway, but nemolizumab is designed to block the signal from a different receptor, the interleukin 31 (IL-31) cytokines. This is the "itch-specific" cytokine, and by targeting this receptor, nemolizumab has been found to effectively reduce the itch caused by eczema.

Results for nemolizumab's phase 2b clinical trial were presented at the annual meeting of the American Academy of Dermatology in March 2019. The trial found that participants on a 30-milligram dose of nemolizumab achieved a 68.8 percent skin improvement at week 24. Nemolizumab has been found to result in rapid and sustained improvements in skin itching in patients with eczema, including improving sleep disturbance and quality of life. It has been found to have an acceptable safety profile.

Nemolizumab has been granted breakthrough therapy designation by the FDA for treating prurigo nodularis, a rare skin disease that is characterized by the formation of hard, itchy nodules on the skin. The breakthrough therapy designation is meant to expedite the development and review of drugs that clinical trials demonstrate may offer substantial improvement over other available therapies. Prurigo nodularis is associated with chronic itching and is frequently found in patients with a history of eczema.

**Etokimab**—This biologic drug targets a different signaling molecule known as interleukin 33 (IL-33), an inflammatory cytokine that is known to play a role in the itch-scratch cycle of eczema. This therapy initially had quite a lot of buzz, but data released from a recent study shows that the drug failed to meet its primary clinical endpoint.

This disappointing finding followed a randomized, double-blind, placebo-controlled study of 300 patients with moderate to severe eczema. The study found no difference in improving eczema symptoms between patients who received an etokimab dose and a placebo. These findings, released in November 2019, throw the future of this drug into doubt, and it could potentially have consequences for other companies hoping to develop IL-33-inhibiting biologics.

**Tezepelumab**—Also known as MEDI9929/AMG 157, this is a fully human monoclonal antibody that inhibits thymic stromal lymphopoietin (TSLP), a protein belonging to the cytokine family that is considered to be a key initiator of allergic inflammation. TSLP is associated not only with eczema but also with asthma. However, some trial studies have found limited efficacy of the drug after 12 weeks of treatment, and findings suggest that future clinical trials may require longer treatment periods.

**GBR 830**—This investigational treatment targets the OX40 cytokine, which is believed to be pivotal in the activation of the Th2 cell skewing in the immune system. Clinical trials of this therapy are ongoing, but there is potential promise that blocking this pathway and reverting the Th2 immune activation could mitigate one of the major causes behind eczema. However, more study is needed.

**Janus Kinase Inhibitors (JAK Inhibitors)**—These drugs are emerging as promising new treatments for many inflammatory conditions, including eczema. They are all given orally and function by inhibiting the activity of one or more of the enzymes in the Janus kinase (JAK) family. These enzymes are JAK1, JAK2, JAK3, and TYK2. It's believed that cytokines signal through JAKs, so blocking JAKs can reduce inflammation associated with eczema. JAK inhibitors are also believed to work on the nerves in the skin and thereby help to mediate itch.

Clinical trials are underway for these drugs, but researchers are getting closer to seeking FDA approval.

- **Tofacitinib**—This drug has been marketed under the brand name Xeljanz and has been approved by the FDA to treat rheumatoid arthritis, ulcerative colitis, and psoriatic arthritis. This JAK inhibitor (which inhibits JAK1 and JAK3) is currently being investigated for use in atopic dermatitis and other conditions. The FDA declined to approve tofacitinib for psoriasis because of safety concerns. The most notable adverse effect was an increased risk of herpes zoster infection, or shingles.

- **Baricitinib**—This drug, which inhibits JAK1 and JAK2, was found to improve eczema in patients with moderate to severe eczema, according to data from a phase 3 study. In a 16-week placebo-controlled trial, the incidence of adverse events and serious adverse events with baricitinib treatment was similar to the placebo; the most common treatment-emergent adverse events observed were the common cold and headache. Other studies also found that using baricitinib along with topical steroids significantly lessened the severity of eczema symptoms in adults.

- **Upadacitinib**—This JAK1 inhibitor significantly improved itch in a recent randomized, placebo-controlled trial enrolling patients with moderate to severe atopic dermatitis. The trial found that, when compared with those in the placebo group, more patients receiving upadacitinib achieved an itch-free state and maintained it over the 16 weeks of the trial. Upadacitinib was approved by the FDA for the treatment of moderate to severe rheumatoid arthritis in August 2019.

- **Abrocitinib**—Some people in the pharmaceutical world believe that this experimental JAK1 inhibitor has a shot at challenging Dupixent as the next blockbuster biologic. The phase 3 study results showed that 62.7 percent of the patients treated with abrocitinib achieved a 75 percent or greater improvement in the severity of their eczema, compared with 11.8 percent in the placebo group. At the twelfth week of treatment, 38.9 percent of the treatment group achieved a 90 percent or greater improvement in their severity scores, versus 5.3 percent of the placebo group.

## GROUNDBREAKING NEW TOPICALS

There are also a number of new topical medications that are being developed and studied through clinical trials. Topical medications are another important way to treat eczema. These treatments can be used in conjunction with other types of medications, or they can be used alone, depending on the severity of the case. These medications can be especially helpful for those patients who don't have severe enough symptoms to warrant taking other types of medications through injection or by mouth.

**Topical JAK Inhibitors**—Researchers are also exploring using JAK inhibitors topically, which could allow patients to apply these medications directly to the site of inflammation and itch, thus minimizing the potential side effects. Because JAK inhibitors are small molecules, they can be applied topically and will penetrate the skin barrier.

Delgocitinib (JTE-052)—This is a topical JAK inhibitor that has been going through clinical trials in Japan. One trial of more than 300 adults, most of whom had moderate atopic dermatitis, found that as the potency of the dose increased, so did the effectiveness of the medication. At a 3 percent dosage, more than 70 percent of the patients saw a reduction in the severity of their eczema symptoms, as well as reduction of itch and very low levels of the medication detected in blood samples.

**Tapinarof**—This drug is a promising topical medication for eczema and the first of its kind: a naturally derived, nonsteroidal anti-inflammatory agent. It activates the aryl hydrocarbon receptor. This leads to a pathway that should reduce both inflammation and itch. Tapinarof has a similar pharmacological function as coal tar. Coal tar therapies have been used for centuries and have been shown to be effective in treating symptoms of eczema. However, they aren't used as often today because they can be messy and smelly. One recent trial for tapinarof showed that about 50 percent of patients with primarily moderate eczema became clear or almost clear when treated twice daily with tapinarof, versus 25 percent of people on a placebo.

# MICROBIOME-BASED TREATMENTS

Another fascinating approach that is very much in its infancy focuses on how strengthening or bolstering the skin's microbiome may help reduce or prevent eczema flares. On a microscopic scale, the skin is a complex ecosystem inhabited by many microorganisms that coexist in an established balance. We know that people with eczema are at much higher risk of developing skin infections and having their skin colonized by an abundance of "bad" bacteria, such as Staphylococcus aureus. During eczema flares, the normal "good" bacteria levels on the skin are greatly reduced, and harmful bacteria take over. This colonization of bad bacteria further drives inflammation and decreases the barrier function of the skin.

Researchers are beginning to look at ways to harness good bacteria to stop bad bacteria from colonizing skin. One recent study looked at culturing good bacteria, such as Staphylococcus hominis, which naturally produces chemicals that kill Staph. aureus bacteria, as a way to topically treat eczema. A small study looked at the therapeutic benefits of using an individual's own good bacteria to counter the bad bacteria on their skin. In this study, swabs were taken from five people and the helpful bacteria, such as Staph. hominis, were cultured and grown and then transplanted back onto active eczema flares. The study showed that the numbers of harmful Staph. aureus plummeted in the first 24 hours after the good bacteria were introduced.

# TOPICAL CANNABINOIDS FOR TREATING ECZEMA

One intriguing area of research that traverses between scientific discovery and natural approaches lies within the science of cannabinoids (chemicals found in cannabis, or marijuana). Topical cannabinoids and endocannabinoids offer another compelling area that appears to have significant potential in dermatology and the treatment of eczema and other inflammatory skin conditions.

Cannabinoids may have anti-inflammatory and anti-itch effects and may offer possible therapies. In several different early trials with patients with eczema, the use of a topical cannabinoid cream was found to help clear mild eczema in 80 percent of patients, decrease the time between flares, and reduce relapses. In another trial, a cream containing the endocannabinoid palmitoylethanolamide (PEA) improved the severity of itch and loss of sleep by an average of 60 percent among subjects. Twenty percent of subjects discontinued their topical immunomodulators, 38 percent ceased using their oral antihistamines, and 33.6 percent no longer felt the need to maintain their topical steroid regimen by the end of the study.

Research and development are still in the early stages, but cannabinoids are a remarkable and diverse group of compounds that may hold significant therapeutic capabilities for eczema.

## THE FUTURE IS BRIGHT

We are living in an exciting era of evolving scientific research. A therapy revolution is underway when it comes to developing new drugs and treatments for eczema. There are many new treatments in the pipeline, and doctors hope many of these will soon be available. But there are still no simple answers, and there is no one easy "cure" that will eliminate eczema for everyone—at least not yet.

"I don't think that there's ever going to be a sort of a magic 'one-size-fits-all' treatment for all of these patients," says Silverberg. "But I do think there are many, many things in the pipeline that we're hopeful about. Wouldn't it be wonderful if we had more options available, so we would be able to get the right drug to the right patient?"

More information is available about investigational drugs or clinical trials for new medications to treat eczema through the US National Library of Medicine website, which maintains an online database on upcoming and ongoing clinical trials in the US: https://clinicaltrials.gov/.

# BIBLIOGRAPHY

## Chapter 1: What's behind Your Itchy, Angry Skin?

American Academy of Dermatology Association. "Atopic Dermatitis: Overview." Accessed September 6, 2019. https://www.aad.org/public/diseases/eczema/types/atopic-dermatitis.

———. "Can You Get Eczema as an Adult?" Accessed September 12, 2019. https://www.aad.org/public/diseases/eczema/adult/can-get.

———. "Nummular Dermatitis: Overview." Accessed September 6, 2019. https://www.aad.org/public/diseases/eczema/types/nummular-dermatitis.

———. "Seborrheic Dermatitis: Overview." Accessed September 6, 2019. https://www.aad.org/public/diseases/scaly-skin/seborrheic-dermatitis.

———. "Stasis Dermatitis: Overview." Accessed September 6, 2019. https://www.aad.org/public/diseases/eczema/types/stasis-dermatitis.

American College of Allergy, Asthma & Immunology. "Eczema in Children." Updated December 28, 2017. https://acaai.org/allergies/who-has-allergies/children-allergies/eczema.

———. "Eczema (Atopic Dermatitis)." Accessed June 1, 2020. https://acaai.org/allergies/types-allergies/skin-allergy/eczema-atopic-dermatitis.

Cleveland Clinic. "Contact Dermatitis." Updated October 10, 2019. https://my.clevelandclinic.org/health/diseases/6173-contact-dermatitis.

Drucker, Aaron M., Annie R. Wang, Wen-Qing Li, Erika Sevetson, and Abrar A. Qureshi. *Audit: Burden of Eczema; The Burden of Disease of Atopic Dermatitis*. San Rafael, CA: National Eczema Association, December 28, 2015. https://nationaleczema.org/wp-content/uploads/2016/06/NEA-report-final12_30_2015.pdf.

Ma, C., J. Stinson, Y. Zhang, et al. "Germline Hypomorphic CARD11 Mutations in Severe Atopic Disease." *Nature Genetics* 49 (June 19, 2017): 1192–1201. https://doi.org/10.1038/ng.3898.

Margolis, J., K. Abuabara, W. Bilker, O. Hoffstad, and D. Margolis. "Persistence of Mild to Moderate Atopic Dermatitis." *JAMA Dermatology* 150, no. 6 (June 2014): 593–600. https://doi.org/10.1001/jamadermatol.2013.10271.

McIntosh, James. "What's to Know about Eczema?" *Medical News Today*, November 14, 2017. https://www.medicalnewstoday.com/articles/14417.

McPherson, T. "Current Understanding in Pathogenesis of Atopic Dermatitis." *Indian Journal of Dermatology* 61, no. 6 (2016): 649–55. https://doi.org/10.4103/0019-5154.193674.

Melina, Remy. "How Much Does Your Skin Weigh?" Live Science, January 13, 2011. https://www.livescience.com/32939-how-much-does-skin-weigh.html.

Nall, Rachel. "What Is the Difference between Nummular Eczema and Ringworm?" *Medical News Today*, August 20, 2018. https://www.medical newstoday.com/articles/322822.

National Eczema Association. "Atopic Dermatitis." Accessed June 1, 2020. https://nationaleczema.org/research/eczema-facts.

National Eczema Association. "Eczema Facts." Accessed March 26, 2020. https://nationaleczema.org/research/eczema-facts.

———. "Dyshidrotic Eczema." Accessed September 6, 2019. https:// nationaleczema.org/eczema/types-of-eczema/dyshidrotic-eczema.

———. "Information and Advice." Accessed March 26, 2020. http://www. eczema.org/information-and-advice.

Thomas, Liji. "Irritant vs Allergic Contact Dermatitis." News-Medical.Net. Accessed September 6, 2019. https://www.news-medical.net/health/ Irritant-vs-Allergic-Contact-Dermatitis.aspx.

Tollefson, M., and A. Bruckner. "Atopic Dermatitis: Skin-Directed Management." *Pediatrics* 134, no. 6 (December 2014): e1735–44. https://doi. org/10.1542/peds.2014-2812.

US National Library of Medicine. "Atopic Dermatitis." Genetics Home Reference. Updated March 17, 2020. https://ghr.nlm.nih.gov/condition/ atopic-dermatitis.

## Chapter 2: Beginning the Healing Process

Ashley Wall (eczema patient advocate, founder of *Itchin Since '87* blog), phone interview with the author, September 12, 2019.

Atherton, D. "Topical Corticosteroids in Atopic Dermatitis." *BMJ* 327, no. 7421 (October 23, 2003): 942–43. https://doi.org/10.1136/bmj.327 .7421.942.

Bennett, Patrick. "Wet Wraps Work Well in Treating Eczema." *Allergic Living*, June 19, 2015. https://www.allergicliving.com/2015/06/19/wet -wraps-work-well-in-treating-eczema.

Crane, Margaret W. "An Old Treatment Approach Offers New Option to Eczema Patients." National Eczema Association. Accessed March 26, 2020. https://nationaleczema.org/old-treatment-new -option-for-eczema.

Danjuma, Zainab (eczema patient advocate and founder of YouTube channel IAmBeeZee), video chat interviews with author, September 9, 2019 and October 11, 2019.

Dolgy, Laura. "What Triggers Eczema? With Dr. Peter Lio." *It's an Itchy Little World*. Updated January 29, 2019. https://itchylittleworld.com/what-triggers-eczema.

Jones, Kathryn. "Everything You Need to Know about Eczema and Food Allergies." National Eczema Association, December 13, 2018. https://nationaleczema.org/eczema-food-allergies.

Kim, InYoung. "Dr. Peter Lio Discusses Integrative Dermatology." *PracticeUpdate*, January 17, 2019. https://www.practiceupdate.com/content/dr-peter-lio-discusses-integrative-dermatology/78618.

Lio, Peter A. "'Natural' Remedies for Eczema: Evidence for the Alternative?" *Practical Dermatology*, February 2013. https://practicaldermatology.com/articles/2013-feb/natural-remedies-for-eczema-evidence-for-the-alternative.

Lio, Peter A. (clinical assistant professor of dermatology and pediatrics at Northwestern University Feinberg School of Medicine and the founding director of the Chicago Integrative Eczema Center), ongoing email interview with author, September 11, 2019 and April 16, 2020.

National Eczema Association. "Education Announcement: Use of Topical Steroids for Eczema." Updated February 8, 2018. https://nationaleczema.org/warnings-for-topical-steroids-eczema.

Rockoff, Alan, and Leslie J. Schoenfield. "A Breakthrough Treatment for Eczema." MedicineNet, June 13, 2018. https://www.medicinenet.com/eczema_a_breakthrough_treatment_for_eczema/views.htm.

US National Library of Medicine. "Hydrocortisone Topical." MedlinePlus. Updated January 15, 2018. https://medlineplus.gov/druginfo/meds/a682793.html.

Woo, T., and P. Kuzel. "Crisaborole 2% Ointment (Eucrisa) for Atopic Dermatitis." *Skin Therapy Letter* 24, no. 2 (March 2019): 4–6.

## Chapter 3: The Basics of Skin Care and Understanding Your Skin

American Academy of Dermatology Association. "What Kids Should Know about the Layers of Skin." Accessed February 27, 2020. https://www.aad.org/public/parents-kids/healthy-habits/parents/kids/skin-layers.

Blicharz, L., L. Rudnicka, and Z. Samochocki. "Staphylococcus Aureus: An Underestimated Factor in the Pathogenesis of Atopic Dermatitis?" *Advances in Dermatology and Allergology* 36, no. 1 (February 2019): 11–17. https://doi.org/10.5114/ada.2019.82821.

Byrd, A., C. Deming, S. Cassidy, O. Harrison, et al. "Staphylococcus Aureus and Staphylococcus Epidermidis Strain Diversity Underlying Pediatric Atopic Dermatitis." July 5, 2017. https://pubmed.ncbi.nlm.nih.gov/28679656.

Chopra, R., P. Vakharia, R. Sacotte, and J. Silverberg. "Efficacy of Bleach Baths in Reducing Severity of Atopic Dermatitis: A Systematic Review and Meta-Analysis." *Annals of Allergy, Asthma & Immunology* 119, no. 5 (November 2017): 435–40. https://doi.org/10.1016/j.anai.2017.08.289.

Cosmetics Info. "Sodium Lauryl Sulfate and Sodium Laureth Sulfate." Accessed April 16, 2020. https://cosmeticsinfo.org/sodium-lauryl-sulfate -and-sodium-laureth-sulfate.

Feuillie, C., P. Vitry, M. McAleer, S. Kezic, A. Irvine, J. Geoghegan, and Y. Dufrêne. "Adhesion of Staphylococcus Aureus to Corneocytes from Atopic Dermatitis Patients Is Controlled by Natural Moisturizing Factor Levels." *MBio* 9, no. 4 (July/August 2018). https://doi.org/10.1128/mbio.01184-18.

Fowler, Joseph. "Understanding the Role of Natural Moisturizing Factor in Skin Hydration." *Practical Dermatology*, July 2012. https://practical dermatology.com/articles/2012-jul/understanding-the-role-of-natural -moisturizing-factor-in-skin-hydration.

Friedman, Adam (interim chair of Dermatology, Residency Program director, director of Translational Research, and director of Supportive Oncodermatology at the George Washington University School of Medicine and Health Sciences), phone interview with author, November 8, 2019.

Gong, J., L. Lin, T. Lin, F. Hao, F. Zeng, Z. Bi, D. Yi, et al. "Skin Colonization by Staphylococcus Aureus in Patients with Eczema and Atopic Dermatitis and Relevant Combined Topical Therapy: A Double-Blind Multicentre Randomized Controlled Trial." *British Journal of Dermatology* 155, no. 4 (October 2006): 680–87. https://doi.org/10.1111/j.1365-2133.2006.07410.x.

Hirsch, Jesse. "How to Find Real Relief for Dry Skin." *Consumer Reports*, April 7, 2019. https://www.consumerreports.org/medical-conditions/find-real -relief-for-dry-skin.

Lee, Margaret. "Basic Skin Care for Eczema: A Dermatologist's Review." National Eczema Association, January 9, 2014. https://nationaleczema.org/ basic-skin-care-eczema.

McCormack, Caitlin. "The Best Cleansing, Non-irritating Soaps for People with Eczema." Everyday Health, August 21, 2018. https://www.everyday health.com/products/reviews/best-cleansing-non-irritating-soaps -for-eczema.

McNamara, Damian. "Tips for Taming Atopic Dermatitis and Managing Expectations." *MDedge Pediatrics*, February 23, 2017. https://www.mdedge. com/pediatrics/article/132025/atopic-dermatitis/ tips-taming-atopic-dermatitis-and-managing-expectations.

Meneghin, F., V. Fabiano, C. Mameli, and G. Zuccotti. "Probiotics and Atopic Dermatitis in Children." *Pharmaceuticals* 5, no. 7 (July 6, 2012): 727–44. https://doi.org/10.3390/ph5070727.

Mohammed, Yousuf. "What Is Sodium Lauryl Sulfate, and Why Are People Avoiding It in Soap and Toothpaste?" *ScienceAlert*, January 7, 2020. https://www.sciencealert.com/this-common-soap-and-toothpaste-chemical-can-be-a-skin-irritant.

Nakatsuji, T., T. Chen, S. Narala, K. Chun, et al.. "Antimicrobials from Human Skin Commensal Bacteria Protect Against Staphylococcus Aureus and Are Deficient in Atopic Dermatitis." *Science Translational Medicine* 9, no. 378 (February 22, 2017). https://pubmed.ncbi.nlm.nih.gov/28228596/.

Paller, A., H. Kong, P. Seed, S. Naik, T. Scharschmidt, R. Gallo, T. Luger, et al. "The Microbiome in Patients with Atopic Dermatitis." *Journal of Allergy and Clinical Immunology* 143, no. 1 (January 2019): 26–35. https://doi.org/10.1016/j.jaci.2018.11.015.

Proksch, E., H. Nissen, M. Bremgartner, and C. Urquhart. "Bathing in a Magnesium-Rich Dead Sea Salt Solution Improves Skin Barrier Function, Enhances Skin Hydration, and Reduces Inflammation in Atopic Dry Skin." *International Journal of Dermatology* 44, no. 2 (February 2005): 151–57. https://doi.org/10.1111/j.1365-4632.2005.02079.x.

Schettle, Lidia, and Peter A. Lio. "Probiotics: The Search for Bacterial Balance." National Eczema Association. Updated January 24, 2018. https://nationaleczema.org/search-bacterial-balance.

Talakoub, Lily, and Naissan O. Wesley. "Probiotic, Prebiotic, and Postbiotic Skin Care." *MDedge Dermatology*, February 13, 2019. https://www.mdedge.com/dermatology/article/194433/aesthetic-dermatology/probiotic-prebiotic-and-postbiotic-skin-care.

Wong, Sam. "Bad Eczema Flare-Ups May Be Caused by Strains of Bacteria." *New Scientist*, July 5, 2017. https://www.newscientist.com/article/2139827-bad-eczema-flare-ups-may-be-caused-by-strains-of-bacteria.

Yirka, Bob. "Study Shows Skin Microbiome Imbalance Likely behind Eczema Flareups." Medical Xpress, May 2, 2019. https://medicalxpress.com/news/2019-05-skin-microbiome-imbalance-eczema-flareups.html.

## Chapter 4: Personal Stories and Strategies for Living Well with Eczema

Lora, Ashley (eczema patient advocate, wellness entrepreneur, founder of VisionHERy), phone interview with author, October 24, 2019.

Roberge, Jennifer (eczema patient caregiver, advocate, and founder of The Eczema Company), phone interview with author, October 23, 2019.

Tapao, Peter (eczema patient advocate, strength and conditioning coach, and group exercise instructor and a personal trainer), phone interviews with author, September 23, 2019 and April 15, 2019.

# Chapter 5: The Link between Eczema and Other Allergic Diseases

Al-Ahmed, Nasser, Shirina Alsowaidi, and Peter Vadas. "Peanut Allergy: An Overview." *Allergy, Asthma & Clinical Immunology*, December 15, 2008. https://doi.org/https://doi.org/10.1186/1710-1492-4-4-139.

American Academy of Allergy, Asthma & Immunology. "Researchers Give New Perspective on Progression from Eczema to Asthma and Allergies." November 15, 2017. https://www.aaaai.org/about-aaaai/newsroom/news-releases/eczema.

American Academy of Allergy, Asthma & Immunology. "Study Gives Insight into What Triggers Cause Anaphylaxis and How Deadly It Is." March 2018. https://www.aaaai.org/about-aaaai/newsroom/news-releases/anaphylaxis.

Balas, K., K. Robbins, M. Jacobs, A. Ramos, D. DiGiacomo, and L. Herbert. "Exclusive Breastfeeding in Infancy and Eczema Diagnosis at 6 Years of Age." *Journal of Allergy and Clinical Immunology* 143, no. 2 (February 2019): AB124. https://doi.org/10.1016/j.jaci.2018.12.377.

Bantz, S., Z. Zhu, and T. Zheng. "The Atopic March: Progression from Atopic Dermatitis to Allergic Rhinitis and Asthma." *Journal of Clinical & Cellular Immunology* 5, no. 2 (April 2014): 1–8. https://doi.org/10.4172/2155-9899 .1000202.

Chang, A., R. Robison, M. Cai, and A. Singh. "Natural History of Children with Food Triggered Atopic Dermatitis and Development of Immediate Reactions." *Journal of Allergy and Clinical Immunology* 135, no. 2 (February 2015): AB264. https://doi.org/10.1016/j.jaci.2014.12.1802.

Chui, Asriani (professor of pediatrics [allergy and immunology] and medicine and director of the Asthma and Allergy Clinic at the Children's Hospital of Wisconsin/Medical College of Wisconsin), ongoing email interviews with author between October 17 and November 4, 2019.

Du Toit, G., G. Roberts, P. Sayre, H. Bahnson, S. Radulovic, A. Santos, H. Brough, et al. "Randomized Trial of Peanut Consumption in Infants at Risk for Peanut Allergy." *New England Journal of Medicine* 372, no. 9 (February 26, 2015): 803–13. https://doi.org/10.1056/nejmoa1414850.

Finkelman, Fred. "Peanut Allergy and Anaphylaxis." *Current Opinion in Immunology* 22, no. 6 (December 2010): 783–88. https://www.ncbi.nlm.nih. gov/pmc/articles/PMC3005304.

Food Allergy Research & Education. "Oral Food Challenge." Accessed March 2, 2020. https://www.foodallergy.org/life-with-food-allergies/food-allergy-101/diagnosis-testing/oral-food-challenge.

Greer, F., S. Sicherer, and A. Burks. "The Effects of Early Nutritional Interventions on the Development of Atopic Disease in Infants and

Children: The Role of Maternal Dietary Restriction, Breastfeeding, Hydrolyzed Formulas, and Timing of Introduction of Allergenic Complementary Foods." *Pediatrics* 143, no. 4 (April 2019). https://doi.org/10.1542/peds.2019-0281.

Gupta, Ruchi (professor of pediatrics and medicine at Northwestern Medicine and director of the Center for Food Allergy & Asthma Research within Northwestern University Feinberg School of Medicine's Institute for Public Health and Medicine), email interview with author, December 11, 2019.

Gupta, Ruchi S. "What about the Food? How Food Can Help or Harm Your Eczema." Webinar Wednesdays. National Eczema Association, December 13, 2018. YouTube video. https://youtu.be/ubKfgpMpnX0.

Gupta, R., C. Lau, E. Sita, B. Smith, and M. Greenhawt. "Factors Associated with Reported Food Allergy Tolerance among US Children." *Annals of Allergy, Asthma & Immunology* 111, no. 3 (September 2013): 194–98. https://doi.org/10.1016/j.anai.2013.06.026.

Gupta, R., C. Warren, B. Smith, J. Blumenstock, J. Jiang, M. Davis, and K. Nadeau. "The Public Health Impact of Parent-Reported Childhood Food Allergies in the United States." *Pediatrics* 142, no. 6 (December 2018). https://doi.org/10.1542/peds.2018-1235.

Gupta, R., C. Warren, B. Smith, J. Jiang, J. Blumenstock, M. Davis, R. Schleimer, et al. "Prevalence and Severity of Food Allergies among US Adults." *JAMA Network Open* 2, no. 1 (January 4, 2019). https://doi.org/10.1001/jamanetworkopen.2018.5630.

Gupta, Ruchi, Robert Sidbury, and Aiden Boomer. "A Closer Look at the Atopic Dermatitis Patient Journey: Effective Management Approaches Across the Age and Disease Spectrum." Accessed April 17, 2020. https://peerview.com/p/index.html?collection=150205756-2&presentation=150205756-2-p1&MemberID=999&Promocode=700#screen1.

Katta, R., and M. Schlichte. "Diet and Dermatitis: Food Triggers." *Journal of Clinical and Aesthetic Dermatology* 7, no. 3 (March 2014): 30–36. https://www.ncbi.nlm.nih.gov/pmc/articles/PMC3970830.

Mayo Clinic. "Seasonal Allergies: Nip Them in the Bud." Mayo Foundation for Medical Education and Research, April 16, 2020. https://www.mayoclinic.org/diseases-conditions/hay-fever/in-depth/seasonal-allergies/art-20048343.

Murdoch Children's Research Institute. "The Five 'Ds' of Food Allergy." May 8, 2015. https://www.mcri.edu.au/news/investigating-allergies-food-allergy-capital.

National Institutes of Health. "Study Finds Peanut Consumption in Infancy Prevents Peanut Allergy." US Department of Health and Human Services,

February 23, 2015. https://www.nih.gov/news-events/news-releases/
study-finds-peanut-consumption-infancy-prevents-peanut-allergy.

Sicherer, Scott H. "New Guidelines Detail Use of 'Infant-Safe' Peanut to
Prevent Allergy." *AAP News*, January 5, 2017. https://www.aappublications
.org/news/2017/01/05/PeanutAllergy010517.

Young, Alex. "Allergies Linked to Increased Risk for Eosinophilic Esophagitis."
*Healio Gastroenterology*, March 5, 2018. https://www.healio.com/
gastroenterology/esophagus/news/online/%7Bf20e503a-cd07-4d5d-94a9-
885a4863c9f9%7D/presence-of-other-allergies-can-predict-eosinophilic
-esophagitis.

## Chapter 6: Holistic and Alternative Treatment Options

American Association of Naturopathic Physicians. "Principles of Naturopathic
Medicine." Accessed March 2, 2020. https://naturopathic.org/page/
PrinciplesNaturopathicMedicine.

American Board of Physician Specialties. "American Board of Integrative
Medicine (ABOIM)." Accessed March 29, 2020. https://www.abpsus.org/
integrative-medicine.

Bonneteau, Rebecca (naturopath, nutritionist, and founder of "The Eczema
Expert"), video interview with author, December 12, 2019.

British Homeopathic Association. "What Is Homeopathy?" Accessed March 2,
2020. https://www.britishhomeopathic.org/homeopathy/what-is
-homeopathy.

Buchkina, Julia. "Introduction to Functional Medicine." The Institute for
Functional Medicine. Accessed March 2, 2020. https://ir.uiowa.edu/cgi/
viewcontent.cgi?article=1085&context=fmrc.

Cameron, Tara (East Asian medicine practitioner specializing in nutrition and
herbal medicine), interview with author, December 27, 2019.

Davis, Stephanie. "Treating Eczema with Functional Medicine: 101." Website
of Dr. Stephanie Davis, February 26, 2018. https://drstephaniedavis.com/
treating-eczema-functional-medicine-101.

Gagné, Claire. "Dr. Li and Her Chinese Herbal Remedies." *Allergic Living*,
December 15, 2015. https://www.allergicliving.com/2015/12/15/dr-li
-and-her-chinese-herbal-remedies.

Goddard, A., and P. Lio. "Alternative, Complementary, and Forgotten
Remedies for Atopic Dermatitis." *Evidence-Based Complementary and
Alternative Medicine* 2015 (July 15, 2015): 1–10. https://doi.org/10.1155
/2015/676897.

Gorick, Robert. "EFT for Skin Problems—Eczema—Rashes." Rob's Hypnosis,
April 13, 2018. YouTube video. https://www.youtube.com/watch?v=
mTkekCtP3Zw.

Hegde, P., D. Hemanth, S. Emmi, M. Shilpa, P. Shindhe, and Y. Santosh. "A Case Discussion on Eczema." *International Journal of Ayurveda Research* 1, no. 4 (October–December 2010): 268–70.

Leonard, Jayne. "A Guide to EFT Tapping." *Medical News Today*, September 26, 2019. https://www.medicalnewstoday.com/articles/326434.

Lio, Peter A. "Alternative Therapies in Atopic Dermatitis Care, Part I." *Practical Dermatology*, June 2011. https://practicaldermatology.com/articles/2011-jun/alternative-therapies-in-atopic-dermatitis-care-part-i.

McMenamy, C., R. Katz, and M. Gipson. "Treatment of Eczema by EMG Biofeedback and Relaxation Training: A Multiple Baseline Analysis." *Journal of Behavior Therapy and Experimental Psychiatry* 19, no. 3 (1988): 221–27. https://doi.org/10.1016/0005-7916(88)90045-6.

Moyer, Krista. "Naturopathic Treatment of Eczema." *Naturopathic Doctor News and Review*, May 5, 2014. https://ndnr.com/dermatology/naturopathic-treatment-of-eczema.

National Ayurvedic Medical Association. "What Is Ayurveda?" Accessed March 2, 2020. https://www.ayurvedanama.org/what-is-ayurveda.

National Center for Complementary and Integrative Health. "Complementary, Alternative, or Integrative Health: What's in a Name?" US Department of Health and Human Services. Updated July 2018. https://www.nccih.nih.gov/health/complementary-alternative-or-integrative-health-whats-in-a-name.

———. "The Use of Complementary and Alternative Medicine in the United States." US Department of Health and Human Services, September 24, 2017. https://www.ncbi.nlm.nih.gov/pmc/articles/PMC2935644/.

National Eczema Association. "Can Meditation Help Ease Eczema Itch?" March 30, 2020. https://nationaleczema.org/meditation-ease-itch.

ScienceDaily. "It's Official—Spending Time Outside Is Good for You." July 6, 2018. https://www.sciencedaily.com/releases/2018/07/180706102842.htm.

Stewart, A., and S. Thomas. "Hypnotherapy as a Treatment for Atopic Dermatitis in Adults and Children." *British Journal of Dermatology* 132, no. 5 (1995): 778–83. https://doi.org/10.1111/j.1365-2133.1995.tb00726.x.

Tabish, S. "Complementary and Alternative Healthcare: Is It Evidence-Based?" *International Journal of Health Sciences* 2, no. 1 (January 2008): v–ix. https://www.ncbi.nlm.nih.gov/pmc/articles/PMC3068720.

Ventola, C. "Current Issues Regarding Complementary and Alternative Medicine (CAM) in the United States." *Pharmacy and Therapeutics* 35, no. 8 (2010): 461–68. https://www.ncbi.nlm.nih.gov/pmc/articles/PMC2935644.

# Chapter 7: Eczema and Nutrition

Bath-Hextall, F., F. Delamere, and H. Williams. "Dietary Exclusions for Improving Established Atopic Eczema in Adults and Children: Systematic Review." *Allergy* 64, no. 2 (February 2009): 258–64. https://doi.org/10.1111/j.1398-9995.2008.01917.x.

Brazier, Yvette. "What Is a Food Intolerance?" *Medical News Today*, December 20, 2017. https://www.medicalnewstoday.com/articles/263965.

Chung, Bo., S. Cho, I. Ahn, H. Lee, H. Kim, C. Park, and C. Lee. "Treatment of Atopic Dermatitis with a Low-Histamine Diet." *Annals of Dermatology* 23, suppl. 1 (September 2011): S91–95. https://doi.org/10.5021/ad.2011.23.s1.s91.

Food Intolerance Network. "Histamine Levels in Food." Updated December 6, 2013. https://www.food-intolerance-network.com/food-intolerances/histamine-intolerance/histamine-levels-in-food.html.

Hadrich, D. "Microbiome Research Is Becoming the Key to Better Understanding Health and Nutrition." *Frontiers in Genetics* 9 (June 13, 2018). https://doi.org/10.3389/fgene.2018.00212.

Hamblin, James. "The Jordan Peterson All-Meat Diet." *Atlantic*, August 28, 2018. https://www.theatlantic.com/health/archive/2018/08/the-peterson-family-meat-cleanse/567613.

Histamine Intolerance Awareness. "The Food List." Accessed March 4, 2020. https://www.histamineintolerance.org.uk/about/the-food-diary/the-food-list.

Lio, Peter. "Leaky Gut, Leaky Skin, or Both?" *Dermatology Times*, May 22, 2019. https://www.dermatologytimes.com/atopic-dermatitis/leaky-gut-leaky-skin-or-both.

———. "Non-Pharmacologic Therapies for Atopic Dermatitis." *Current Allergy and Asthma Reports* 13, no. 5 (October 2013): 528–38. https://doi.org/10.1007/s11882-013-0371-y.

Migala, Jessica. "On the Carnivore Diet, People Are Eating Only Meat: Here's What to Know." EverydayHealth, September 10, 2018. https://www.everydayhealth.com/diet-nutrition/diet/carnivore-diet-benefits-risks-food-list-more.

Phan, C., M. Touvier, E. Kesse-Guyot, M. Adjibade, S. Hercberg, P. Wolkenstein, O. Chosidow, et al. "Association between Mediterranean Anti-Inflammatory Dietary Profile and Severity of Psoriasis." *JAMA Dermatology* 154, no. 9 (September 2018): 1017–24. https://doi.org/10.1001/jamadermatol.2018.2127.

Sissons, Beth. "What Are the Benefits of Quercetin?" *Medical News Today*, January 14, 2019. https://www.medicalnewstoday.com/articles/324170.

Thompson, M., and J. Hanifin. "Effective Therapy of Childhood Atopic Dermatitis Allays Food Allergy Concerns." *Journal of the American Academy of Dermatology* 53, no. 2, suppl. 2 (August 2005): S214–19. https://doi.org/10.1016/j.jaad.2005.04.065.

UW Integrative Health. "The Elimination Diet." University of Wisconsin–Madison School of Medicine and Public Health, November 2018. https://www.fammed.wisc.edu/files/webfm-uploads/documents/outreach/im/handout_elimination_diet_patient.pdf.

Worm, M., E. Fiedler, S. Dölle, T. Schink, W. Hemmer, R. Jarisch, and T. Zuberbier. "Exogenous Histamine Aggravates Eczema in a Subgroup of Patients with Atopic Dermatitis." *Acta Dermato-Venereologica* 89, no. 1 (2009): 52–56. https://doi.org/10.2340/00015555-0565.

Yaghoobi, R., A. Kazerouni, and O. Kazerouni. "Evidence for Clinical Use of Honey in Wound Healing as an Anti-bacterial, Anti-inflammatory Antioxidant and Anti-viral Agent: A Review." *Jundishapur Journal of Natural Pharmaceutical Products* 8, no. 3 (August 2013): 100–4. https://www.ncbi.nlm.nih.gov/pubmed/24624197.

## Chapter 8: Everyday Natural Approaches to Treating Eczema

Araújo, C., J. Gomes, A. Vieira, F. Ventura, J. Fernandes, and C. Brito. "A Proposal for the Use of New Silver-Seaweed-Cotton Fibers in the Treatment of Atopic Dermatitis." *Cutaneous and Ocular Toxicology* 32, no. 4 (2013): 268–74. https://doi.org/10.3109/15569527.2013.775655.

Dayrit, F. "The Properties of Lauric Acid and Their Significance in Coconut Oil." *Journal of the American Oil Chemists' Society* 92, no. 1 (January 2015): 1–15. https://doi.org/10.1007/s11746-014-2562-7.

*Dermatology Times.* "Manuka Honey Tested as AD Treatment." October 6, 2017. https://www.dermatologytimes.com/eczema-treatments/manuka-honey-tested-ad-treatment.

Fowler, J., J. Nebus, W. Wallo, and L. Eichenfield. "Colloidal Oatmeal Formulations as Adjunct Treatments in Atopic Dermatitis." *Journal of Drugs in Dermatology* 11, no. 7 (July 2012): 804–7. https://www.ncbi.nlm.nih.gov/pubmed/22777219.

Gray, N., A. Dhana, D. Stein, and N. Khumalo. "Zinc and Atopic Dermatitis: A Systematic Review and Meta-Analysis." *Journal of the European Academy of Dermatology and Venereology* 33, no. 6 (June 2019): 1042–50. https://doi.org/10.1111/jdv.15524.

Huotari, Anne, and Karl-Heinz Herzig. "Vitamin D and Living in Northern Latitudes—an Endemic Risk Area for Vitamin D Deficiency." *International Journal of Circumpolar Health* 67, no. 2–3 (June 2008): 164–78. https://doi.org/10.3402/ijch.v67i2-3.18258.

Irani, Mahboubeh, Marziyeh Sarmadi, Francoise Bernard, Gholam Hossein
Ebrahimi Pour, and Hossein Shaker Bazarnov. "Leaves Antimicrobial
Activity of Glycyrrhiza Glabra L." *Iranian Journal of Pharmaceutical
Research* 9, no. 4 (2010): 425–28. https://www.ncbi.nlm.nih.gov/pmc/articles/
PMC3870067.

Jones, Kathryn. "Get the Facts: Apple Cider Vinegar." National Eczema
Association, December 13, 2018. https://nationaleczema.org/get-facts-acv.

Kalliomäki, M., S. Salminen, H. Arvilommi, P. Kero, P. Koskinen, and E.
Isolauri. "Probiotics in Primary Prevention of Atopic Disease: A
Randomised Placebo-Controlled Trial." *Lancet* 357, no. 9262 (April 7, 2001):
1076–79. https://doi.org/10.1016/s0140-6736(00)04259-8.

Kasprowicz, Sarah. "Tea Tree Oil: What Can It Do for Your Patients?"
*Dermatology Times*, August 11, 2015. https://www.dermatologytimes.com/
editors-choice-derm/tea-tree-oil-what-can-it-do-your-patients.

Lio, Peter A. "'Natural' Remedies for Eczema: Evidence for the Alternative?"
*Practical Dermatology*, February 2013. https://practicaldermatology.com/
articles/2013-feb/natural-remedies-for-eczema-evidence-for-the-alternative.

———. "The Irregular Border." *Dermatology Times*, February 8, 2015. https://
www.dermatologytimes.com/dermatology/irregular-border.

Mlcek, J., T. Jurikova, S. Skrovankova, and J. Sochor. "Quercetin and Its
Anti-Allergic Immune Response." *Molecules* 21, no. 5 (May 2016). https://doi.
org/10.3390/molecules21050623.

Nall, Rachel. "Can Tea Tree Oil Treat Eczema?" *Medical News Today*, June 11,
2018. https://www.medicalnewstoday.com/articles/322103.

Saeedi, M., K. Morteza-Semnani, and M. Ghoreishi. "The Treatment of Atopic
Dermatitis with Licorice Gel." *Journal of Dermatological Treatment* 14, no. 3
(2003): 153–57. https://doi.org/10.1080/09546630310014369.

Shi, K., and P. Lio. "Alternative Treatments for Atopic Dermatitis: An Update."
*American Journal of Clinical Dermatology* 20, no. 2 (April 2019): 251–66.
https://doi.org/10.1007/s40257-018-0412-3.

Sidbury, R., A. Sullivan, R. Thadhani, and C. Camargo. "Randomized
Controlled Trial of Vitamin D Supplementation for Winter-Related Atopic
Dermatitis in Boston: A Pilot Study." *British Journal of Dermatology* 159, no.
1 (July 2008): 245–47. https://doi.org/10.1111/j.1365-2133.2008.08601.x.

Thomas, K., L. Bradshaw, T. Sach, J. Batchelor, S. Lawton, E. Harrison, R.
Haines, et al. "Silk Garments plus Standard Care Compared with Standard
Care for Treating Eczema in Children: A Randomised, Controlled,
Observer-Blind, Pragmatic Trial (CLOTHES Trial)." *PLOS Medicine* 14, no.
4 (April 11, 2017). https://doi.org/10.1371/journal.pmed.1002280.

Varma, S., T. Sivaprakasam, I. Arumugam, N. Dilip, M. Raghuraman, K.
Pavan, M. Rafiq, et al. "*In Vitro* Anti-inflammatory and Skin Protective

Properties of Virgin Coconut Oil." *Journal of Traditional and Complementary Medicine* 9, no. 1 (January 2019): 5–14. https://doi.org/10.1016/j.jtcme.2017 .06.012.

Weston, S., A. Halbert, P. Richmond, and S. Prescott. "Effects of Probiotics on Atopic Dermatitis: a Randomised Controlled Trial." *Archives of Disease in Childhood* 90, no. 9 (September 2005): 892–97. https://doi.org/10.1136/ adc.2004.060673.

Yaghoobi, R., A. Kazerouni, and O. Kazerouni. "Evidence for Clinical Use of Honey in Wound Healing as an Anti-Bacterial, Anti-Inflammatory Anti-Oxidant and Anti-Viral Agent: A Review." *Jundishapur Journal of Natural Pharmaceutical Products* 8, no. 3 (August 2013): 100–104.

Zhu, Z., Z. Yang, C. Wang, and H. Liu. "Assessment of the Effectiveness of Vitamin Supplement in Treating Eczema: A Systematic Review and Meta-Analysis." *Evidence-Based Complementary and Alternative Medicine* 2019 (October 31, 2019): 1–10. https://doi.org/10.1155/2019/6956034.

## Chapter 9: Burning Skin and Topical Steroids

Arnold, K., A. Treister, and P. Lio. "Dupilumab in the Management of Topical Corticosteroid Withdrawal in Atopic Dermatitis: A Retrospective Case Series." *JAAD Case Reports* 4, no. 9 (October 2018): 860–62. https://doi. org/10.1016/j.jdcr.2018.06.012.

Banos, Briana (eczema patient advocate, documentary film producer of *Preventable: Protecting Our Largest Organ*), phone interview with author, September 16, 2019.

Banos, Briana, dir. *Preventable: Protecting Our Largest Organ*. March 22, 2019. https://preventabledoc.com.

Barclay, Laurie. "Use of Topical Corticosteroids for Dermatologic Conditions Reviewed." Medscape, January 21, 2009. https://www.medscape.org/ viewarticle/587108.

Hajar, T., Y. Leshem, J. Hanifin, S. Nedorost, P. Lio, A. Paller, J. Block, et al. "A Systematic Review of Topical Corticosteroid Withdrawal ('Steroid Addiction') in Patients with Atopic Dermatitis and Other Dermatoses." *Journal of the American Academy of Dermatology* 72, no. 3 (March 2015): 541–49. https://doi.org/10.1016/j.jaad.2014.11.024.

Hyams, J., and D. Carey. "Corticosteroids and Growth." *Journal of Pediatrics* 113, no. 2 (August 1988): 249–54. https://doi.org/10.1016/s0022-3476(88) 80260-9.

ITSAN. "About ITSAN." Accessed March 26, 2020. https://www.itsan .org/about-itsan.

Jancin, Bruce. "SDEF: Contact Allergy to Corticosteroid—The Stealth Allergy." *MDedge*, March 19, 2010. https://www.mdedge.com/dermatology/article/11229/pediatrics/sdef-contact-allergy-corticosteroid-stealth-allergy.

Kristmundsdottir, F., and T. J. David. "Growth Impairment in Children with Atopic Eczema." *Journal of the Royal Society of Medicine* 80, no. 1 (January 1987): 9–12. https://journals.sagepub.com/doi/pdf/10.1177/014107688708000106.

Li, A., E. Yin, and R. Antaya. "Topical Corticosteroid Phobia in Atopic Dermatitis." *JAMA Dermatology* 153, no. 10 (October 2017): 1036–42. https://doi.org/10.1001/jamadermatol.2017.2437.

Lio, Peter A., and Neha Chandan. "Topical Steroid Withdrawal in Atopic Dermatitis." *Practical Dermatology*, August 2009. https://practical dermatology.com/articles/2019-aug/topical-steroid-withdrawal-in-atopic -dermatitis.

National Collaborating Centre for Women's and Children's Health (UK). *Atopic Eczema in Children: Management of Atopic Eczema in Children from Birth up to the Age of 12 Years*. NICE Clinical Guidelines, no. 57. London: RCOG Press, 2007. https://www.ncbi.nlm.nih.gov/books/NBK49354.

Ozdemir, A., and V. Bas. "Iatrogenic Cushing's Syndrome Due to Overuse of Topical Steroid in the Diaper Area." *Journal of Tropical Pediatrics* 60, no. 5 (October 2014): 404–6. https://doi.org/10.1093/tropej/fmu036.

Pace, W. "Topical Corticosteroids." *Canadian Medical Association Journal* 108, no. 1 (January 6, 1973): 11–13. https://www.ncbi.nlm.nih.gov/pmc/articles/PMC1941119/pdf/canmedaj01659-0013.pdf.

Robertson, Sally. "Steroid Induced Rosacea." News-Medical.Net, August 23, 2018. https://www.news-medical.net/health/Steroid-Induced-Rosacea.aspx.

Sathishkumar, Dharshini, and Celia Moss. "Topical Therapy in Atopic Dermatitis in Children." *Indian Journal of Dermatology* 61, no. 6 (November 2016): 656–61. https://doi.org/10.4103/0019-5154.193677.

Sheary, B. "Steroid Withdrawal Effects Following Long-Term Topical Corticosteroid Use." *Dermatitis* 29, no. 4 (July/August 2018): 213–18. https://doi.org/10.1097/der.0000000000000387.

Silverberg, Jonathan (professor of dermatology, director of clinical research, and director of patch testing for the George Washington University School of Medicine's Department of Dermatology), phone interview with author, January 24, 2020.

## Chapter 10: Treating Eczema in Skin of Color

Alexis, Andrew. "Eczema in Skin of Color: What You Need to Know." Webinar Wednesdays. National Eczema Association, September 26, 2019. YouTube video. https://youtu.be/_0pCqykKBYo.

Alexis, Andrew (director of the Skin of Color Center at Mount Sinai West in New York. He is also the chair of the Department of Dermatology at Mount Sinai West and professor of dermatology at the Icahn School of Medicine at Mount Sinai), phone interview with author, February 20, 2020.

Centers for Disease Control and Prevention. "QuickStats: Percentage of Children Aged ≤17 Years with Eczema or Any Kind of Skin Allergy, by Selected Races/Ethnicities—National Health Interview Survey, United States, 2000–2010." Morbidity and Mortality Weekly Report (MMWR), November 11, 2011. https://www.cdc.gov/mmwr/preview/mmwrhtml/mm6044a9.htm.

Fischer, A., D. Shin, D. Margolis, and J. Takeshita. "Racial and Ethnic Differences in Health Care Utilization for Childhood Eczema: An Analysis of the 2001-2013 Medical Expenditure Panel Surveys." *Journal of the American Academy of Dermatology* 77, no. 6 (December 2017): 1060–67. https://doi.org/10.1016/j.jaad.2017.08.035.

Genetic and Rare Diseases Information Center. "Prurigo Nodularis." US Department of Health and Human Services. Updated April 19, 2018. https://rarediseases.info.nih.gov/diseases/7480/prurigo-nodularis.

HealthDay News. "Prurigo Nodularis More Likely in African-Americans." *Clinical Advisor*, September 14, 2018. https://www.clinicaladvisor.com/home/dermatology/prurigo-nodularis-more-likely-in-african-americans.

Jungersted, J., J. Høgh, L. Hellgren, G. Jemec, and T. Agner. "Ethnicity and Stratum Corneum Ceramides." *British Journal of Dermatology* 163, no. 6 (December 2010): 1169–73. https://doi.org/10.1111/j.1365-2133.2010.10080.x.

Muizzuddin, N., L. Hellemans, L. Van Overloop, H. Corstjens, L. Declercq, and D. Maes. "Structural and Functional Differences in Barrier Properties of African American, Caucasian and East Asian Skin." *Journal of Dermatological Science* 59, no. 2 (August 1, 2010): 123–28. https://doi.org/10.1016/j.jdermsci.2010.06.003.

Mutasim, Diya F. "What Is Psoriasiform Dermatitis?" In *Practical Skin Pathology*, 23–25. Cham, Switzerland: Springer, 2015.

Noda, S., M. Suárez-Fariñas, B. Ungar, S. Kim, C. de Guzman Strong, H. Xu, X. Peng, et al. "The Asian Atopic Dermatitis Phenotype Combines Features of Atopic Dermatitis and Psoriasis with Increased TH17 Polarization." *Journal of Allergy and Clinical Immunology* 136, no. 5 (November 2015): 1254–64. https://doi.org/10.1016/j.jaci.2015.08.015.

Sanyal, R., A. Pavel, J. Glickman, T. Chan, X. Zheng, N. Zhang, I. Cueto, et al. "Atopic Dermatitis in African American Patients Is TH2/TH22-Skewed with TH1/TH17 Attenuation." *Annals of Allergy, Asthma & Immunology* 122, no. 1 (January 2019): 99–110. https://doi.org/10.1016/j.anai.2018.08.024.

Wesley, N., and H. Maibach. "Racial (Ethnic) Differences in Skin Properties." *American Journal of Clinical Dermatology* 4, no. 12 (December 2003): 843–60. https://doi.org/10.2165/00128071-200304120-00004.

## Chapter 11: Eczema's Impact on Mental Health and Overall Well-Being

American Academy of Allergy, Asthma & Immunology. "Atopic Eczema Linked to Increased Risk of Cardiovascular Disease." December 18, 2018. https://www.aaaai.org/global/latest-research-summaries/Current-JACI-Research/cardiovascular.

"Atopic Dermatitis in America Study Overview." *Atopic Dermatitis in America Study Overview*. Arlington, VA: Asthma and Allergy Foundation of America in partnership with the National Eczema Association, 2018. https://www.aafa.org/media/2209/Atopic-Dermatitis-in-America-Study-Overview.pdf.

Ascott, A., A. Mulick, A. Yu, D. Prieto-Merino, M. Schmidt, K. Abuabara, L. Smeeth, et al. "Atopic Eczema and Major Cardiovascular Outcomes: A Systematic Review and Meta-Analysis of Population-Based Studies." *Journal of Allergy and Clinical Immunology* 143, no. 5 (May 2019): 1821–29. https://doi.org/10.1016/j.jaci.2018.11.030.

Chernyshov, P. "Stigmatization and Self-Perception in Children with Atopic Dermatitis." *Clinical, Cosmetic, and Investigational Dermatology* 9 (2016): 159–66. https://doi.org/10.2147/ccid.s91263.

"Facts & Statistics." Anxiety and Depression Association of America, ADAA. Accessed April 17, 2020. https://adaa.org/about-adaa/press-room/facts-statistics.

Gamse, Caroline. "Atopic Dermatitis Hikes Risk of Autoimmune Disorders." Medpage Today, April 5, 2019. https://www.medpagetoday.com/resource-centers/spotlight-pediatric-atopic-dermatitis/atopic-dermatitis-hikes-risk-autoimmune-disorders/2473.

Jeon, C., D. Yan, M. Nakamura, S. Sekhon, T. Bhutani, T. Berger, and W. Liao. "Frequency and Management of Sleep Disturbance in Adults with Atopic Dermatitis: A Systematic Review." *Dermatology and Therapy* 7, no. 3 (September 2017): 349–64. https://doi.org/10.1007/s13555-017-0192-3.

Kantor, Robert, Ashley Kim, Jacob Thyssen, and Jonathan Silverberg. "Association of Atopic Dermatitis with Smoking: A Systematic Review and Meta-Analysis." *Journal of the American Academy of Dermatology* 75, no. 6 (December 2016): 1119–25. https://doi.org/10.1016/j.jaad.2016.07.017.

Koo, J., and A. Lebwohl. "Psychodermatology: The Mind and Skin Connection." *American Family Physician* 64, no. 11 (December 2001): 1873–79. https://www.aafp.org/afp/2001/1201/p1873.html.

Narla, S., and J. Silverberg. "Association between Atopic Dermatitis and Autoimmune Disorders in US Adults and Children: A Cross-Sectional Study." *Journal of the American Academy of Dermatology* 80, no. 2 (February 2019): 382–89. https://doi.org/10.1016/j.jaad.2018.09.025.

Panovska, V. "Anxiety and Depression in Family Members and Caregivers of Preschool Children with Atopic Dermatitis." *EMJ Dermatology* 7, no. 1 (2019): 60–61. https://www.emjreviews.com/dermatology/abstract/anxiety-and-depression-in-family-members-and-caregivers-of-preschool-children-with-atopic-dermatitis.

Penn Medicine. "Not Just for Children: Study Shows High Prevalence of Atopic Dermatitis among U.S. Adults." Penn Medicine News, October 30, 2018. https://www.pennmedicine.org/news/news-releases/2018/october/not-just-for-children-study-shows-high-prevalence-of-atopic-dermatitis-among-us-adults.

Roesner, Lennart M., and Thomas Werfel. "Autoimmunity (or Not) in Atopic Dermatitis." *Frontiers in Immunology* 10 (September 10, 2019). https://doi.org/10.3389/fimmu.2019.02128.

Sandhu, J., K. Wu, T. Bui, and A. Armstrong. "Association between Atopic Dermatitis and Suicidality." *JAMA Dermatology* 155, no. 2 (February 2019): 178–87. https://doi.org/10.1001/jamadermatol.2018.4566.

Silverberg, J., J. Gelfand, D. Margolis, M. Boguniewicz, L. Fonacier, M. Grayson, P. Ong, et al. "Symptoms and Diagnosis of Anxiety and Depression in Atopic Dermatitis in U.S. Adults." *British Journal of Dermatology* 181, no. 3 (September 2019): 554–65. https://www.ncbi.nlm.nih.gov/pubmed/30838645.

Silverberg, Jonathan, and Philip Greenland. "Eczema and Cardiovascular Risk Factors in 2 US Adult Population Studies." *The Journal of Allergy and Clinical Immunology* 135, no. 3 (March 2015): 721–28.

Strom, M., A. Fishbein, A. Paller, and J. Silverberg. "Association between Atopic Dermatitis and Attention Deficit Hyperactivity Disorder in U.S. Children and Adults." *British Journal of Dermatology* 175, no. 5 (November 2016): 920–29. https://doi.org/10.1111/bjd.14697.

Zuberbier, T., S. Orlow, A. Paller, A. Taïeb, R. Allen, J. Hernanz-Hermosa, J. Ocampo-Candiani, et al. "Patient Perspectives on the Management of Atopic Dermatitis." *Journal of Allergy and Clinical Immunology* 118, no. 1 (July 2006): 226–32. https://doi.org/10.1016/j.jaci.2006.02.031.

## Chapter 12: The Era of Eczema: New Therapies on the Horizon

Dermira, Inc. "Dermira Receives Fast Track Designation from FDA for Lebrikizumab for the Treatment of Atopic Dermatitis." Business Wire,

December 10, 2019. https://www.businesswire.com/news/home/2019
1210005383/en.

Dotinga, Randy. "VIDEO: With New Therapies Available, It's the 'Decade of
Eczema,' Researcher Says." *MDedge Dermatology*, February 23, 2018.
https://www.mdedge.com/dermatology/article/159303/atopic-dermatitis/
video-new-therapies-available-its-decade-eczema.

Ernst, Diana. "Baricitinib Added to Topical Steroids Beneficial in Atopic
Dermatitis Trial." MPR, September 3, 2019. https://www.empr.com/home/
news/drugs-in-the-pipeline/baricitinib-added-to-topical-steroids-beneficial
-in-atopic-dermatitis-trial.

Fleming, P. "Tofacitinib: A New Oral Janus Kinase Inhibitor for Psoriasis."
*British Journal of Dermatology* 180, no. 1 (January 2019): 13–14. https://doi.
org/10.1111/bjd.17323.

Friedman, Adam. "Cannabinoids in Dermatology." *Practical Dermatology*,
March 8, 2018. https://practicaldermatology.com/meeting-coverage/
san-diego-2018-feb/cannabinoids-in-dermatology.

GlobalData Healthcare. "Future of IL-33 Inhibition in Atopic Dermatitis in
Doubt." Clinical Trials Arena, November 15, 2019. https://www.
clinicaltrialsarena.com/comment/future-of-il-33-inhibition-in-atopic
-dermatitis-in-doubt.

*Healio Dermatology*. "Baricitinib Meets Primary Endpoint in Adults with
Atopic Dermatitis." August 26, 2019. https://www.healio.com/dermatology/
dermatitis/news/online/%7B91bf00e0-a1b0-4a28-8717-1712d5e6b9e8%7D/
baricitinib-meets-primary-endpoint-in-adults-with-atopic-dermatitis.

———. "Oral Upadacitinib Monotherapy Significantly Improves Eczema
Severity." December 12, 2019. https://www.healio.com/dermatology/
dermatitis/news/online/%7Bcfc0b587-3e66-4d21-ae99-3487041426d4%7D/
oral-upadacitinib-monotherapy-significantly-improves-eczema-severity.

———. "Researchers Explore Potential of Cannabinoids in Inflammatory,
Neoplastic Skin Diseases." May 3, 2019. https://www.healio.com/
dermatology/dermatitis/news/online/%7B0ffd4339-e73d-4a8f-a55a-
15c0a7118ad4%7D/researchers-explore-potential-of-cannabinoids-in
-inflammatory-neoplastic-skin-diseases.

Jancin, Bruce. "Once-Daily Oral JAK Inhibitor for Atopic Dermatitis Effective
in Phase 3 Study." *MDedge Dermatology*, October 18, 2019. https://www.
mdedge.com/dermatology/article/210418/atopic-dermatitis/once-daily
-oral-jak-inhibitor-atopic-dermatitis.

———. "Topical Tapinarof Heads for Phase 3 in Atopic Dermatitis and
Psoriasis." *MDedge Rheumatology*, November 11, 2017. https://www
.mdedge.com/rheumatology/article/151783/psoriasis/topical-tapinarof
-heads-phase-3-atopic-dermatitis-and.

Nakagawa, H., O. Nemoto, A. Igarashi, and T. Nagata. "Efficacy and Safety of Topical JTE-052, a Janus Kinase Inhibitor, in Japanese Adult Patients with Moderate-to-Severe Atopic Dermatitis: A Phase II, Multicentre, Randomized, Vehicle-Controlled Clinical Study." *British Journal of Dermatology* 178, no. 2 (February 2018): 424–32. https://doi.org/10.1111/bjd.16014.

Nakatsuji, T., T. Chen, S. Narala, K. Chun, A. Two, T. Yun, F. Shafiq, et al. "Antimicrobials from Human Skin Commensal Bacteria Protect against *Staphylococcus Aureus* and Are Deficient in Atopic Dermatitis." *Science Translational Medicine* 9, no. 378 (February 22, 2017). https://doi.org/10.1126/scitranslmed.aah4680.

Nygaard, U., C. Vestergaard, and M. Deleuran. "Emerging Treatment Options in Atopic Dermatitis: Systemic Therapies." *Dermatology* 233, no. 5 (February 2018): 344–57. https://doi.org/10.1159/000484406.

Paller, Amy. "Era of Eczema—Treatments in Development." Webinar Wednesdays. National Eczema Association, March 8, 2018. YouTube video. https://youtu.be/2wvnXLg_jgQ.

Renert-Yuval, Y., and E. Guttman-Yassky. "New Treatments for Atopic Dermatitis Targeting beyond IL-4/IL-13 Cytokines." *Annals of Allergy, Asthma & Immunology* 124, no. 1 (January 2020): 28–35. https://doi.org/10.1016/j.anai.2019.10.005.

Sanofi. "Sanofi: Dupixent® (Dupilumab) Showed Positive Topline Results in Phase 3 Trial of Children Aged 6 to 11 Years with Severe Atopic Dermatitis." GlobeNewswire News Room, August 6, 2019. https://www.globenewswire.com/news-release/2019/08/06/1897265/0/en/Sanofi-Dupixent-dupilumab-showed-positive-topline-results-in-Phase-3-trial-of-children-aged-6-to-11-years-with-severe-atopic-dermatitis.html.

Shalaby, Michael, Helena Yardley, and Peter A. Lio. "Stirring the Pot: Cannabinoids and Atopic Dermatitis." *Practical Dermatology*, January 2018. https://practicaldermatology.com/articles/2018-jan/stirring-the-pot-cannabinoids-and-atopic-dermatitis.

Silverberg, N., and J. Silverberg. "Inside Out or Outside In: Does Atopic Dermatitis Disrupt Barrier Function or Does Disruption of Barrier Function Trigger Atopic Dermatitis?" *Cutis* 96, no. 6 (December 2015): 359–61. https://www.ncbi.nlm.nih.gov/pubmed/26761930.

Simpson, E., J. Parnes, D. She, S. Crouch, W. Rees, M. Mo, and R. van der Merwe. "Tezepelumab, an Anti-Thymic Stromal Lymphopoietin Monoclonal Antibody, in the Treatment of Moderate to Severe Atopic Dermatitis: A Randomized Phase 2a Clinical Trial." *Journal of the American*

*Academy of Dermatology* 80, no. 4 (April 2019): 1013–21. https://doi.org/
10.1016/j.jaad.2018.11.059.

Smith, S., C. Jayawickreme, D. Rickard, E. Nicodeme, T. Bui, C. Simmons, C.
Coquery, et al. "Tapinarof Is a Natural AhR Agonist that Resolves Skin
Inflammation in Mice and Humans." *Journal of Investigative Dermatology*
137, no. 10 (October 2017): 2110–19. https://doi.org/10.1016/j.jid.2017.05.004.

Taylor, Nick Paul. "Pfizer Posts Detailed Phase 3 Data on Its Dupixent Rival."
FierceBiotech, October 12, 2019. https://www.fiercebiotech.com/biotech/
pfizer-posts-detailed-phase-3-data-its-dupixent-rival.

US Food and Drug Administration. "FDA Approves Eucrisa for Eczema." FDA
Newsroom, December 14, 2016. https://www.fda.gov/news-events/press-
announcements/fda-approves-eucrisa-eczema.

# INDEX

## A

Abrocitinib, 203
acupuncture, 100
adrenal insufficiency, 154
air, 98
Alexis, Andrew, 163–169, 172, 174
Allen, Katie, 76
allergen, 71–72
allergic contact dermatitis, 17
 sources, 17
 symptoms, 18
allergic diseases/reactions and
 eczema, 69–90
 allergic rhinitis (hay fever), 69
 antihistamines, 72
 decongestants, 72
 environmental allergies, 69–70, 72
 food allergies, 69, 73–75
 foods, 72
 insect stings, 72
 itch, 71–73
 latex, 72
 link between, 70–71
 medications, 72
 nasal sprays, 72
 reasons for becoming, 76–77
 sneezing, 71–73
 swelling, 71–73
allergic rhinitis (hay fever), 69
allergy antibody testing, 85–86
allergy skin test, 87
 intradermal skin test, 87
 skin prick test, 87
all-meat diet, 125
aloe vera gel, 29
alternative medicine, 94–95

alternative treatment options, 97–102.
 *See also* Traditional Chinese
 Medicine (TCM)
 ayurveda, 97, 98–99
 growing trend, 92–93
 homeopathy, 97, 98
 naturopathy, 97
 reasons for, 93
 remedies, 97
alternative treatments, validity of,
 109–111
American Academy of Pediatrics
 (AAP), 79
American Association of
 Naturopathic Physicians, 97
American Board of Physician
 Specialties (ABPS), 95
anaphylaxis, 72, 83, 86
angry skin. *See* itchy skin
antibacterial therapy, 29
anxiety
 eczema and, 103, 176
 as eczema symptom, 180–181
apple cider vinegar, 30, 138–139
Aron, Richard, 29
Asthma and Allergy Foundation of
 America, 72
atopic dermatitis (AD), 16
atopic eczema, 32
atopic march (allergic march), 65,
 69–71, 90
attention deficit hyperactivity
 disorder (ADHD), 179–180
autoimmune disorders, eczema's
 impact on, 186–187
avascular necrosis of femoral head,
 154

fighting eczema naturally, 29–30. *See also* natural treatments

integrative approaches, 23

mind and body therapies, 31

mind-body practices, 23

mindset practice, 59–62

self-diagnosis, 24

heart disease and eczema, 187

herpes simplex, 50

high-histamine foods, 122–123

histamine-liberating foods, 122–123

holistic health practitioners, 95–96. *See also* practitioners

holistic treatment options, 91–111

conventional methods and, 96

food to heal, 108

nutrition to heal, 108

principles, 94

reconnecting with nature, 108–109

homeopathy, 97, 98

honey, 30, 130–131

humectants, 48

hydrocortisone, 26, 151

hyperpigmentation, 169, 172–173

hyperreactive immune system, 13flare-ups, 13–14

hypersensitivity reaction, 34

hypertrichosis, 153

hypnotherapy, 103

hypopigmentation, 153

**I**

iatrogenic Cushing's syndrome, 154

immune system, eczema's impact on, 186–187

immunoglobulin E (IgE) antibodies, 81, 85

inattentiveness, eczema and, 179–180

inflamed skin, 6

"inside out" theory, 193–194

integrative approach in treatments, 30

integrative medicine, 95

intensity, 88

interleukin 4 (IL-4), 196

interleukin 13 (IL-13), 196

interleukin 31 (IL-31), 200

interleukin 33 (IL-33), 201

International Study of Life with Atopic Eczema, 177–178

International Topical Steroid Addiction Network (ITSAN), 145, 155

intestinal hyperpermeability. *See* leaky gut syndrome

intradermal skin test, 87

irritant contact dermatitis, 17

itch, 71–73

itchiness, 12–21, 178–179

"itch-scratch-itch" cycle, 37–38

itchy skin, 12–21

causing agents, 13

risky people, 14–15

**J**

Janus kinase (JAK) inhibitors, 202–203

baricitinib, 202–203

tofacitinib, 202

upadacitinib, 203

**L**

Lack, Gideon, 77

lactobacillus, 51

leaky gut syndrome, 113–115

leaky skin, 195

Learning Early About Peanut Allergy (LEAP), 78

lebrikizumab, 199–200

lesions, 166–167

Li, Xiu-Min, 99

lichen planus, 168

lichenification, 152

lichenoid variant, 168

licorice root extract, 135–136

light therapy, 28–29

hurdles to, 25
hydrocortisone, 26
to mend hard-to-heal skin, 25–29
moisturizer use, 25
new options, 27–29
nonsteroidal medicines, 27–29
oral steroids, 27
second-line treatment, 28–29
systemic immunosuppressants, 28
topical steroids, 26–27
triamcinolone, 151
trigger for eczema, 31–34
atopic eczema, 32
chronic eczema, 32
identifying, 33
trigger, food as, 35–37
types of eczema, 15–21, 24. *See also*
contact dermatitis
atopic dermatitis (AD), 16
dyshidrotic eczema, 20
nummular eczema, 19–20
stasis dermatitis, 21

**V**

Validated Investigator Global
Assessment scale for Atopic
Dermatitis (vIGA-AD scale), 89
vaseline, 49
vedic culture of India, 98
venous eczema. *See* stasis dermatitis
venous stasis dermatitis. *See* stasis
dermatitis
vicious cycle, breaking, 37–38

viral infections, 50
vitamin D, 76, 133–134

**W**

water, 98
well-balanced diet, 127
wet wrapping, 27, 139–140
wheat-free diets, 126–127
wool, 141
working through eczema, 106–107
chronic eczema, 107
mental impact, 107
mind and spirit, 107
trauma linked to, 106–107
wraps, 139–141
dry wrapping, 140
keeping eczema under, 139–141
wet wrapping, 139–140

**X**

Xeljanz, 202

# ACKNOWLEDGMENTS

Much of this book is based on the research and insight provided by a number of knowledgeable sources who deal with eczema on a personal or professional level every day. Their voices, experience, and wisdom are woven into this book, and I couldn't have written it without them.

I am deeply grateful to Dr. Peter Lio, Dr. Adam Friedman, Dr. Asriani Chiu, Dr. Ruchi Gupta, Dr. Andrew Alexis, and Dr. Jonathan Silverberg, who all took time out of their busy schedules to answer questions and provide valuable medical information into the management, treatment, and ongoing research into eczema. They also helped me understand some of the deeper issues pertaining to this skin disorder and its connections to other conditions. This book relies heavily on the wealth of knowledge they shared. I'd also like to give a special thanks to Dr. Lio, whose boundless expertise on this topic helped me discern and synthesize medical research and information used in many areas throughout this book.

I am also deeply appreciative of the insight and knowledge shared by the alternative practitioners interviewed for this book. I spoke at length with Rebecca Bonneteau, a naturopathic practitioner, and Tara Cameron, an East Asian medicine practitioner, and they were both invaluable in illuminating how holistic and alternative medicine seeks to treat the whole patient (not just the skin), and also helped me better understand the fundamental philosophies behind these modalities. I also want to thank Jennifer Roberge, founder of The Eczema Company and blog, *It's an Itchy Little World*. Roberge's deep understanding